"Pina shares the master keys to capturing the elegant glow that we crave."

—Mehmet Oz, MD

"Dr. LoGiudice has written a very helpful book that provides a gold mine of proven, safe, and affordable techniques for inner and outer beauty. Her entertaining writing style is well reasoned, clear, and easy to understand, but does not skimp on the science. The prescriptive advice is also first-rate. Her 'little book' is in fact a giant contribution to the science of self-care."

—Peter D'Adamo, ND, author of
Eat Right for Your Type

"We all know that eating right and exercising are imperative for our overall health, but often we don't realize that what we apply to our skin directly impacts our health as well. If you're looking to create a healthy beauty routine with lasting and unparalleled results, then *The Little Book of Healthy Beauty* is the resource for you. Your beauty routine doesn't have to be toxic or boring; in fact this guide will show you that natural beauty is not only healthier but more effective and ultraglamorous as well!"

—Marissa Waller, founder and curator of
BeauTeaBar, Inc.

The
LITTLE BOOK
of
HEALTHY
BEAUTY

Simple Daily Habits to
Get You Glowing

PINA LOGIUDICE, ND, LAC

A TARCHERPERIGEE BOOK

tarcherperigee

An imprint of Penguin Random House LLC
375 Hudson Street
New York, New York 10014

Most TarcherPerigee books are available at special quantity discounts for bulk purchase for sales promotions, premiums, fund-raising, and educational needs. Special books or book excerpts also can be created to fit specific needs. For details, write: SpecialMarkets@penguinrandomhouse.com.

ISBN 9780399176937

Printed in the United States of America
3   5   7   9   10   8   6   4   2

Book design by Elke Sigal

*This book is dedicated to all who have come to me
for care. Thank you for the privilege to walk with you
on your health journey. I have learned so much.*

*And to Peter and Sophia,
you are my life, my peace, and my joy.*

CONTENTS

INTRODUCTION

My mom, Carmela, seventy-one years old as of this writing, is my inspiration to keep healthy and defy aging. She is an active gardener and artist—she started watercolor painting in her early sixties—and as a grandmother of seven, she gets down and dirty, giving hugs, chasing kids, and laughing with love. Born in Sicily, she lives the Mediterranean diet (with no short supply of olive oil, garlic, and fresh vegetables every day) and has been a marvel to her prescribing doctors by using exercise and supplements, instead of pharmaceuticals, to work her way out of osteoporosis. Her skin looks great, and her mind is sharp. She really exemplifies matriarchal wisdom and strong, supportive love (and she makes the best cannoli on the planet).

In comparison, some patients I work with come in for their first visit using a walker, barely making it out of the car and to the door of my office. By age seventy, they look like they are in their eighties. Why is it that some people age gracefully and stay strong while others look twice their age, even at forty?

INTRODUCTION

Welcome! I'm Dr. Pina LoGiudice (pronounced "lo-JUDY-chay"). I'm honored that you're letting me guide you to your most vibrant health and glow. You are reading this book possibly because you are interested in learning about health and want to create a healthier and more vibrant you. Or it could be because you are facing some health challenges and would like a practical guide to helping your body begin to heal itself. Either way, this will be a great place for you to start.

A Little About Me

Many of you may have seen me as one of the go-to natural doctors on *The Dr. Oz Show* but have wondered who I am and what my background is. Well, in short, I'm a naturopathic doctor and a licensed acupuncturist. I studied at the National Institutes of Health, where I researched stress and the mind-body connection before going to a medical school that focuses on holistic and integrative care. If you haven't heard of a naturopathic doctor, you will. We're the doctors of the future. The philosophy of naturopathic medicine is to combine excellent science-based care with the most natural methods to help the body *heal itself.* I believe all medicine has its place, and that the best doctors know how to properly integrate (but not overuse) conventional medicine such as drugs and surgery with natural healing for the best patient care possible.

After medical school, I started my practice in New York with my husband, Dr. Peter Bongiorno, where we have been working with patients for the past eleven years, using the principles that you and I are going to go over together in this book. One thing Peter and I learned in medical school is that the word *doctor* comes from the Latin verb *docere*, which means "to teach." It is every doctor's job (and my privilege) to do just that.

And now it is my honor to teach you how to reach your best health. You and I will spend our time together understanding sleep, foods, lifestyle, exercise, and natural remedies such as vitamins and herbs. Having come into natural medicine due to my own health crisis, I understand the circuitous journey to health. Thank God pioneering doctors introduced me to natural medicine and to some of the concepts in this book. Those concepts turned my life around and made a major challenge a learning triumph. I am so glad to have the opportunity to share this work with you.

What Do I Mean by Glow?

So, what does it mean to glow? When I talk about "glow," I'm really just trying to articulate that almost indescribable but obvious radiance, beauty, and energetic vitality exuded by people who are truly healthy and happy. This kind of glow can't be created with makeup, and it isn't born in a plastic surgeon's office.

The glow I have in mind is undeniable. It is the kind of radiance that naturally emanates from a young child. It is the look that communicates vitality, essence, and energy. It is also what a gracious and elegant senior exudes if she is vital and vibrant. Glow doesn't have an age limit—that is, unless you fail to nurture and nourish it.

Unfortunately, our glow is being dimmed despite our advanced technology and medicine. Life expectancy is shortening. A 2005 *New England Journal of Medicine* study showed for the first time that babies born that year would not live as long as their parents. Why would that be? Well, the majority of reasons has to do with what we eat, whether we smoke, and our environment and lifestyle. The good news is that these are all things over which we have great control.

My hope is that with the information in this book, not only are you going to become more vital, but you will have fun in the process. In my own journey to health, I learned that being healthy is not the opposite of having fun. In fact, eating good food and taking great care of yourself are actually more fun and open you up to new experiences, tastes, and sensations. And as you feel better and better, you will find that life is best when you feel your best.

You can experience your best glow with much less effort than you think. This book will explain how.

The Master Keys to Glow

....

In the past eleven years, with the help of my patients, I have developed a program that brings together all I've learned through my research and clinical experience. I have pored over studies, separating the proven and safe from the junk. Moreover, working with many, many patients over this time, I have seen firsthand what works and what doesn't. The six master keys I'm about to share with you represent what is needed for healthy beauty. They are the basics for really glowing. Together, chapter by chapter, we're going to explore each one so that you can unlock your best health.

So let's get started! The six master keys to health, longevity, and glow are:

- Sleep
- Food
- Exercise
- Relaxation
- Detoxification
- Supplement Support

With these, you'll be well on your way.

Navigating This Book and Testing Your Glow Dimmers

···

My hope is that this book will be a fun, accessible read. Much of it will be as easy as pie. However, there will be places where I'll give a little extra, more technical information—the ✳ symbol will indicate when we are diving into the science a little further. If it's too much information, feel free to skip these sections; you will still get the information you need. However, if you are a science geek like me, you'll love these passages. If you are even hungrier for the science and research involved in glowing, you will find plenty of references at the end of the book that lead to the information I discuss.

To get going, there is going to be a test! Don't worry, this is an easy one—it is really just a little quiz to learn up front what your greatest challenges may be. This quiz is designed to help you identify the basic factors that are dimming your glow, so you can focus on the chapters that are right for you to help you find your best vitality.

Each of the following six sections has eight questions. Answer each with a simple yes or no. At the bottom of each set, count the yes responses. Then start your plan with the chapter that corresponds to the highest number of yes answers. For example, if the detoxification section gives you seven yeses, the digestion section gives you four, and sleep gives you three, while the others are zeros, then hit chapter 5 (the detox chapter) first, then move on to chapter 2 (food and digestion) and then chapter 1 (sleep). If a given section gets no yeses from you, then you can skip it, or go over it last. Once you have read all the chapters you need, then go to chapter 7 and write down your personalized glow recommendation list.

Ready, set, glow!

Section 1 — Your Beauty Sleep

1. Do you sleep fewer than 7 hours a night? _____

2. Do you get to bed after 11:00 p.m.? _____

3. Do you have trouble falling asleep? _____

4. Do you have trouble staying asleep? _____

5. Are you a "night owl," feeling more awake in the evening hours? _____

6. Do you have sleep apnea? _____

7. Do people say you look tired? _____

8. Do numerous anxious thoughts jump around your brain at night? _____

Number of yes responses _____

Section 2 ✑ Food and Digestion

1. Do you have fewer than one bowel movement a day? _____

2. Does your digestive system bother you in some way (constipation, diarrhea, bloat, gas, pain, reflux) most days? _____

3. Do you get angry or irritable if you miss a meal (do you feel hungry plus angry, aka "hangry")? _____

4. Do you have days when you don't eat green plant foods? _____

5. Do you drink less than 40 ounces of water a day? _____

6. Do you purchase larger-size clothes and/or put on a pound or more every year or two? _____

7. Is most of your food cooked in someone else's kitchen? _____

8. Do you eat foods cooked at high temperature (e.g., chips or fried foods) every day? _____

Number of yes responses _____

Section 3   *Move in Your Glow Zone*

1. Do you avoid exercise or anything that involves breaking a sweat? _____

2. Are some parts of your body much weaker than others? _____

3. Do you carry excess fat around your stomach, upper arms, butt, or thighs? _____

4. Is walking up steps a chore? _____

5. Is it hard to get up off a couch or chair? _____

6. Are you unable to do a push-up? _____

7. Is your home on one level, with no steps? _____

8. Do you sit for the majority of the day? _____

Number of yes responses _____

Section 4   *Relaxation and Inner Peace*

1. Do you feel negative or anxious most of the time and/or do you hate your work or daily life? _____

2. Do you feel a deep disconnect from other people that makes you feel alone and/or do you consistently feel you are not "good enough"? _____

3. Do you have zero exposure to a park or outdoor space with trees and plants once a day? _____

4. Is meditation, acupuncture, or massage absent from your regularly scheduled life? _____

5. Do you get together with friends, a religious group, or other community less than once a week? _____

6. Is there no time in your life to help other people? _____

7. If someone else is doing well, do you feel there's less for you? _____

8. Do you consider your body "not good looking" and/or will you not look at your naked body in the mirror? _____

Number of yes responses _____

Section 5 ✑ Detoxification

1. Do perfumes and aromas bother you? _____

2. Does a cup of coffee or alcoholic drink make you feel pretty bad or keep you up at night? _____

3. Have you had or do you have regular exposure to pollution and/or chemicals such as those in hair products? _____

4. Do you have age/liver spots on your skin? _____

5. Do you smoke or take medications regularly? _____

6. Do you look older or weigh more than you think you should? _____

7. Does every day involve eating some form of cow's milk, gluten, or meat? _____

8. Do you think you don't sweat, no matter how hard you exercise? _____

Number of yes responses _____

Section 6 ✑ Glowing Supplements and Hormonal Harmony

1. Do you take a quality multiple vitamin fewer than five days a week? _____

2. Do you take essential fatty acids fewer than five days a week? _____

3. Do you take a probiotic supplement fewer than five days a week? _____

4. Do you have menstrual irregularity or perimenopausal/menopausal symptoms? _____

5. Do you miss a rainbow color (red, orange, yellow, green, blue, violet) in your regular diet? _____

6. Does your skin have no shine or luster or is your tongue coat patchy or a little swollen? _____

7. Do you swell or have mood changes, terrific hunger, or insomnia that is affected by your menstrual cycle? _____

8. Are your nails soft, thin, brittle, or furrowed or do you have dry mouth corners? _____

Number of yes responses _____

Now write down in descending order the sections with the most yeses. Read this book in that order, to get started on the areas that need the most attention!

Proof That the Master Keys Work: Epigenetics

Now that you have taken the quiz, you have a good idea about the areas in which you will need the most support. The short chapters in this book will help guide you to ultimate health by using your own body's mechanism to make the most of your genetic information.

Epigenetics is an exciting but not well-known field of genetic research. Our genes are made up of deoxyribonucleic acid (DNA for short). DNA makes up the codes in each of our cells. These codes are basically instructional blueprints so that our bodies know how to be healthy. The field of epigenetics looks at how lifestyle, diet, and environment can control our genes to do their healthy best.

The word *epigenetic* literally means "above the gene." This exciting field shows us that the molecules floating in our body's cells, around our genes, help decide whether a particular gene gets turned on or off. Epigenetic research shows us that 70 percent of genes are controlled by diet, lifestyle, and environment.

Each chapter in this book will help you make better choices in terms of these factors and create a new you as you take your own journey of health. It is an absolute honor to be walking with you on your health and beauty journey. I wish you many years of glow.

Many blessings and great health.

Dr. Pina

The
LITTLE BOOK
of
HEALTHY
BEAUTY

Chapter 1

YOUR BEAUTY SLEEP

Sleep is the golden chain that binds health and
our bodies together.

—THOMAS DEKKER, AUTHOR

*A*ll the makeup in the world isn't going to hide the fact that you're not sleeping. There's a reason it's called "beauty sleep"—and like anger, stress, and bitterness, fatigue shows on your face. Lack of sleep can lead to weight gain, digestive problems, impatience, stress, a sense of being overwhelmed, and an inability to think clearly. Even the U.S. government has officially recognized that lack of sleep can increase vulnerability to major diseases, including high blood pressure, diabetes, depression, and cancer. In 2014 the Centers for Disease Control, which had found that almost one in five people had trouble sleeping, deemed lack of sleep a "public epi-demic."

Yet what if sleeping well isn't simple for you? What if you lie there unable to fall asleep? What if you're able to fall asleep but can't stay asleep? Help is here.

First, let me say a few words about your sleep schedule, because not having a sleep routine is often at the core of a number of sleep issues.

Your Sleep Schedule

In 1640 the poet George Herbert said, "An hour of sleep before midnight is worth three after." That tenet is almost four hundred years old, but it remains true today. At the core of Herbert's bit of wisdom is the fact that the later you go to bed, the less chance your body has to do its necessary repair and anti-inflammatory work. You late owls are wondering, "But what if I go to bed late and sleep in late? Is that just as good?"

No. Unfortunately, it isn't.

As the sun goes down, your body recognizes that the time to sleep is growing near. When your eyes sense darkness, the small pineal gland at the base of your brain begins to release melatonin, the hormone for sleep and the master hormone that sets your body clock. So, maybe it's 8:30 or 9:00 at night and you start to feel a little drowsy. If you wind down the evening and slip under the covers by 10:00 or 10:30, your body naturally continues the "closing up shop for the night" process that began with the lowering of the sun. When you interrupt this natural order of things, however, maybe by watching television or surfing the Internet, you create a stress response and elevate your stress hormone, cortisol. An animal that stays up past dark usually has a desperate need to find food, or to run for its life. Either way, the creature is stressed! Most likely, what feels like a second wind to you is actually your primitive brain thinking, "Wake up! There's trouble!" Do you see how this can impede your ability to wind down and go to sleep?

Okay, now let's try to fix the most common sleep problems.

Sleep Problem 1: "I Can't Fall Asleep"

You're looking forward to bed. You're ready for bed. You crawl into bed. And then you just lie there, wide awake, not even tired—or, worse, wide awake and exhausted. Let's look at some of the possible cures for that life troll insomnia.

Aim for a Bedtime Between 10:30 and 11:00 p.m.

If you go to bed very late, try slowly to inch your bedtime ten to fifteen minutes earlier a week. Such gradual change shouldn't be difficult for your body to adjust to. If you do find it difficult, some natural supplements should help a bit (we'll discuss these under

"Sleep Problem 2"), but try these rituals first, and you may find you won't need the supplements.

Start a Bedtime Ritual One Hour Before Bed

Turn off the bright lights, TV, computer, phone, and tablet. Bright blue light suppresses your natural melatonin, so consider buying an orange bulb for a dedicated lamp, and read a book (yes, a real book, not a lighted electronic one) by that light *only*. Orange light doesn't suppress melatonin as much as regular white light does. Make a small cup of chamomile or lavender tea and sip it slowly. You are becoming verrry sleeeepy . . .

Assess Your Nest

There's an old saying that the bedroom is for sex and sleep. So make sure your boudoir isn't cluttered with extraneous distractions (such as a TV or a computer). Also, how much light is in the bedroom when you're trying to sleep? While I know some people who could sleep through Disney World's Main Street Electrical Parade, many of us are sensitive even to low levels of light and would be well served by blackout shades. An eye mask can help, too—I love the comfy padded ones filled with lavender or flax seeds. Use the hand test: if your room is dark but you can still see your hand twelve inches in front of your face, there's too much light in the room.

Feng Shui for Better Sleep

In Chinese medicine, when your environment is cluttered, your body's energy gets cluttered, too, and unhealthy. Feng shui is the art of organizing your environment so your body's energy flows best. Consider having a feng shui expert check the room to see if anything is getting in the way of good sleeping energy (such as stuff under the bed, too many books, electromagnetic fields, or the bed's position in the room). Better bedroom energy may mean better sleep. There are many wonderful books on the topic.

Here are some more steps my patients have taken successfully to get back into the sleeping groove. Try the first one and give it a few days. If that doesn't work, try the next one.

Starbucked? Cut the Caffeine

I know this hurts—I confess, I'm drinking an early morning soy latte while writing these words—but when I had my insomnia issues, I said good-bye to the caffeine for a few months until my body clock was reset. While caffeine may not be the root cause of a sleeping problem, working with patients has taught me that it's almost impossible to correct sleep issues when there's caffeine in the system. Once you're sleeping again, you have my blessing to do a nice big swan dive into your beloved mochaccino.

If cutting the coffee really hurts (I mean, *really* hurts), then congratulations! You are addicted to caffeine (and right where Starbucks wants you). You know this because when you stop caffeine, your body tells you all about it with whopping headaches, extreme fatigue, and sometimes constipation and even depression.

The fact is it's good to take time away from anything that starts to run you. Try this: Start taking a good, potent B complex in the morning. (It will make your urine very yellow; this is normal.) Also, take 250 milligrams (mg) of magnesium glycinate once a day at bedtime. These two vitamins will minimize the caffeine withdrawal symptoms. Once you have these in your system for a day or two, start the weaning process: For week one, make your coffee three-quarters caffeinated and one-quarter decaffeinated. Week two, move to half-caffeinated and half-decaffeinated. Then, for week three, try one-quarter caffeinated and three-quarters decaffeinated. Finally, for the last week, move to all decaf (which still has a little caffeine in it). After this last week, you should be able to move to an herbal tea such as rooibos, or to Teeccino, a delicious chicory coffee substitute that contains no caffeine.

Avoid Certain Foods Before Bed

Sometimes eating too close to bedtime will also keep you up. When you keep your digestive system up and working late, it can be hard to get the brain to shut down. And here's a little bad news: dark chocolate is another no-no at bedtime, as it easily has enough caffeine to perk you up at the wrong time. Alcohol is confusing because it can help you drop into sleep quickly, but then it disturbs your deeper sleep later by working to stimulate the nervous system. So what felt like a nice buzz will soon morph into a thrashing sleep. Spicy and fatty foods can rile your stomach enough to stop you from sleeping. For optimal slumber, try to put a good three hours between your last meal of the day and your bedtime.

Try Pre-Sleep Sweating

For years the medical community thought exercise close to bedtime was too invigorating and kept people awake at night. Then, in 2013, the National Sleep Foundation found that exercise at any time of day can help people sleep well at night and stay healthier overall. Only 3 percent of late exercisers in the study reported that their sleep was worse after exercise. So exercise when you can and see how it feels for you. More than likely it will help you sleep better.

Quiet Your Mind

Sometimes "racing thoughts" are what keep people awake. Unfortunately we often can't just turn them off. I suggest trying to displace your broken record with a thought, a word, a mantra of some kind. You might silently think of a word or phrase such as "Sleep . . . now." As you breathe in, hear yourself think, "Sleeeeeeeep." As you breathe out, hear "Nowwww." Try to establish a slow, gentle breathing pattern. If you force yourself to repeat a short sequence of words, it's very difficult for other thoughts to push their way in.

Fool Yourself into Feeling Light-Headed

I know a woman who has a bizarre-sounding insomnia cure, but she swears by it, so I think it's worth mentioning. She "daydreams" herself into what feels like the light-headed or drugged state she remembers experiencing before going into surgery: those floaty seconds while she was being anesthetized and starting to float into la-la land. She concentrates on revisiting or re-creating that sensation. Sometimes this involves her focusing on the moving patterns she can observe even though her eyes are closed: fluids and lightness against the darkness behind her eyelids. She claims that fooling herself into thinking she's been given a sedative works every time.

Hug Yourself

Renowned psychologist Elisha Goldstein teaches about mindfulness and offers practical strategies for calming the mind. He teaches a very simple "self-hugging" technique that can also work as a sleep aid. While lying in bed, bend the elbow of one arm and lay that arm across your chest, resting your hand on your opposite shoulder. Then wrap your other arm around your waist. This creates a gentle binding sensation, not unlike the coziness that a snugly swaddled infant feels—and a sense of snugness can help lead to sleep.

Sleep Problem 2: "I Fall Asleep, but Can't Stay Asleep"

Maybe you do try to keep a good sleep schedule and you can fall asleep, but you can't remain asleep for long. Try this trick I keep up my sleeve:

Take Tryptophan

Found naturally in turkey and bananas, this amino acid helps your brain produce more serotonin, which will help you stay peacefully asleep. German studies from the late 1980s showed benefits, but unfortunately the advent of sleep medications curtailed the study of many natural supplements, so more studies have not been completed. I find supplemental tryptophan quite helpful for patients. Try 500 to 2,000 mg. I recommend the product Tryptophan Calmplete, which is dosed from one to four capsules a night.

If tryptophan is not enough, add a little time-released melatonin. For this, I recommend Melatonin Cadence, which is in tablet form. One tablet is 3 mg. Start with half a tablet—they are scored and easily split into two halves—and move up to two full tablets, if needed, to stay asleep. See the "Resources" section at the back of this book for information on finding these supplements.

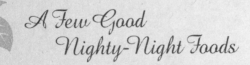

A Few Good Nighty-Night Foods

Often people wake up due to hunger because their liver isn't releasing enough sugar at night to keep them feeling sated until morning. Eating a little food before bed can prevent this. *A little food*. Too much food can keep you awake. You might want to try one of these sleep starters:

Oatmeal

This is one of my favorite nighty-night foods because it contains small amounts of melatonin, the brain chemical that tells your body it's time for bed. Oatmeal is a cereal grain made from the herb

Avena sativa. *Avena sativa* is known in traditional herbal medicine as a calming plant that is nutritious for a frazzled nervous system. Oats contain complex carbohydrates that can help deliver more tryptophan to the brain to help you sleep. They also contain B_6, a vitamin that helps produce serotonin in the brain. Have a quarter cup at bedtime. (If you have issues with constipation, feel free to add a tablespoon of ground flax meal.)

Montmorency cherries

The Montmorency is a special variety of cherry with even more melatonin than its regular old cherry counterpart we see in most supermarkets. You can find these bright red cherries in some fine food stores when they are in season. They can also be found in the frozen section, or look for a Montmorency cherry juice concentrate.

Pumpkin seeds

These have extra tryptophan, which turns into serotonin (a molecule you need to sleep) and then into melatonin in the brain.

Dandelion greens

Dark green leafy vegetables have more nutrients than we will probably ever know. While dandelion greens are not traditionally known as a sleep-inducing food, I have found their liver-cleansing properties to be a valuable sleep aid.

Pulque

Still relatively unfamiliar to most people, pulque is a thousand-year-old native Mexican milk-colored alcoholic beverage made from the fermented sap of the maguey plant (a type of agave), and it is high in melatonin. It is a bit frothier and less alcoholic than its modern beer counterpart. While it is an age-old drink, it is becoming quite popular these days. Thanks to pulque's melatonin and alcohol content, it functions as a relaxant, so it's best to drink it after dinner. It should not be used by anyone with a history of or tendency toward alcoholism, and it should not be ingested by minors or pregnant women. I don't recommend drinking pulque as a daily solution—just an occasional one.

Sleep Problem 3: "I'm Anxious and Need Anxiety Meds to Sleep"

This is quite common. Do sleep medications such as Ambien (zolpidem) or antianxiety meds such as Ativan (lorazepam) and Xanax (alprazolam) help you fall asleep or stay asleep? If your answer is yes, this suggests that your brain is in stress overdrive. You need to calm that brain down.

Basically, your brain has two modes that run simultaneously. One mode deals with the outside, *conscious* world; this is the part of the brain that makes decisions, leads you to action, and is aware of what's happening right now. Then there's the other side, which is more internal. It's your *unconscious*, and it houses your all-important background thoughts, your spirit, your psychic processors. In Chinese medicine there's yang and yin—each of these opposing energies needs a little of the other to be what it is. If you look at the familiar yin-yang illustration, in the white, yang part, there is always a little yin. In the black, yin part, there is always a little yang. Your brain works the same. Even in the daytime (the yang part of the day) your brain needs some yin. (For a picture of yin and yang and a more detailed explanation of this concept, please visit www.drpinaND.com/yinyang.)

Translation: if you haven't managed to connect with your unconscious, spiritual side during the day, it will stand up straight at night and shout, "Okay, *now* you're going to pay attention to me!"—keeping you up. If you think this is part of what's keeping you awake, try one or more of the following:

Write Down What's on Your Mind

Before bed, jot down (by the light of your orange lightbulb) what's on your mind. It needn't be more than bullet points:

- I'm worried about Mom's health.
- I really dislike that new girl at work.
- I wish I hadn't yelled at my daughter.
- Do I have enough wine and cheese for the dinner party?

As some writers say, "I write to figure out what I think." Some people view writing as a conversation with themselves. Having this kind of quick conversation before sleep might help you put some thoughts to bed right along with you.

Make a To-Do List

Simple as that. Sometimes, if you feel overwhelmed by everything you have to accomplish, organizing, producing, managing, and *conquering* a to-do list can spare you the pressure of mentally cycling through the countless details. The physical act of writing them down can ease your mind.

Once you've done this, though, set the list aside and take comfort in the fact that it's all right there, on paper. You're not going to forget anything, and you don't have to deal with it now. It can wait until tomorrow.

Check Your Hormones

If all these sleep tips aren't launching you into sweet dreams, ask your naturopathic physician for an adrenal stress panel, a simple test that involves spitting into a small tube four times a day to check your hormones and circadian rhythms. Also consider blood work to check estrogen and progesterone levels. Many of my patients in their thirties, forties, and fifties have experienced progesterone decline (which can be exacerbated by stress and poor diet). When progesterone is low, the GABA system drops out. GABA stands for "gamma-aminobutyric acid," a neurotransmitter that places your brain in calm mode. If your progesterone is low, you might be a candidate for progesterone supplements, which are extremely safe and can even protect against hormonal cancers such as those of the breast and uterus. For sleep, progesterone supplements are usually dosed by mouth at bedtime. They help naturally raise GABA and calm the mind.

A Word About Sleeping Pills

People often ask me, "Why shouldn't I just take a sleep medication?" Indeed, it's a popular solution; roughly nine million people in the United States take them every night. Most sleeping pill users are in their fifties or older, but in the past twenty years, younger people have tripled their use of sleep aids.

While sleeping pills can make people fall asleep and stay asleep, it's merely a surface sleep, one that doesn't let the body run the healing processes it needs to run. As a result, these pills can cause health issues. A 2012 *British Medical Journal* study of thirty thousand subjects found a more than threefold increased risk of death in people taking a dose of sleeping pills eighteen times a year (which averages to not even two pills a month). The risk shot up to five times when the pills were taken more often—which is concerning, because most patients take them every night.

If you are taking sleep medication, the best thing is to discuss this concern with your prescribing doctor and look for a practitioner well versed in natural methods to help you sleep.

Instead of Drugs . . .

Your body knows how to fall asleep, and natural methods can help bring you proper rest. Here are two beautiful brain calmers you can take quite effectively instead of drugs. You might try just one, or even both together if needed. Talk to your doctor before stopping your medications. Please remember that if you are on medication, you should *never* stop abruptly to try natural methods. Let your prescribing doctor know of your interest in natural medicines to see what is safe for you. It is not smart to jump on and off drugs. That can cause more harm to your body and mind.

GABA (Gamma-Aminobutyric Acid)

A personal favorite, GABA is a naturally occurring amino acid the brain uses to stay calm and relaxed. Low GABA levels are associated with insomnia. Supplemental GABA has been shown to be an effective relaxant and helps relieve anxiety. Start with one 500 mg capsule at bedtime; you can go up to 1,000 mg if needed. GABA is best taken on an empty stomach, to maximize absorption.

Passionflower (Passiflora)

This herb is great for the mind that runs in circles and won't shut down. With its calming flavonoids and alkaloids, it's been as effective as Ativan in people with generalized anxiety disorder—but without the side effects of, say, an SSRI (selective serotonin reuptake inhibitor) such as Lexapro (escitalopram). Passionflower is thought to raise your levels of GABA naturally, to relax you into a nice, natural slumber. It has even been shown to lower anxiety before dental work, so it must be good. You can take passionflower in tea, capsule, or liquid form. I typically prescribe thirty drops of the liquid (called a tincture) in a small glass of water before bedtime. This wonderful plant medicine will help you wake up feeling refreshed and beautiful in the morning.

Some Q&A on R&R

....

Here are a few questions I am often asked on the subject of sleep.

I always hear that people should get at least eight hours of sleep a night. What if I feel fine with six?

Getting fewer than seven hours of sleep a night has been shown to leave us 300 percent more likely to catch common viruses and get sick. Ask yourself the following: Could my energy level be higher? Do I get sick more often than I should? Do I have sugar and food cravings? Do I have trouble losing weight? If any of these deliver a yes, you may want to try seven to eight hours of sleep to see if it makes you feel better than you do now.

Why do older people seem to need less sleep? Why do they like to get up earlier?

A United Kingdom study a few years back showed that as we age, we can function and stay alert after less sleep than we used to need. People in their late sixties to eighties can easily tolerate forty to sixty minutes less sleep than twenty- and thirtysomethings. Research has also shown that seniors spend less time in a deep sleep, which is likely why they tend to awaken earlier.

There are so many "natural" teas that claim to be sleep aids. Do any of them work?

They do work well. My favorite sleep tea contains valerian. This herb is the most researched for sleep and has a natural Xanax-like effect by raising the level of calming neurotransmitters in your brain. My second favorite is lavender, which works nicely for those who have trouble calming down. Another tasty favorite is schizandra, also known as wu wei zi, a delicious berry that the Chinese have used for thousands of years for people whose stress keeps them up at night.

Is there value in napping? Can I nap for too long?

Short naps (twenty to thirty minutes) a few times a week have been linked to lower rates of heart disease and the boosting of brain function throughout the rest of the day. If you have the luxury, I say go for it, but try not to nap for more than a half hour. After thirty minutes, you may drop into a sleep deep enough to impact your nighttime rhythm negatively. According to a 2014 *American Journal of Epidemiology* report, long naps of an hour or more are even associated with dying sooner. (Yikes!) So nap regularly but keep it under thirty minutes and do it before 3:00 p.m.

If I have vivid, frequent, or long dreams, does that mean I'm sleeping well?

Some vivid dreaming can be normal. I believe most dreaming is an attempt by your unconscious to figure things out that might be challenging for you—and that's a good thing. Vivid dreams occur during a more wakeful part of your sleep, called REM (rapid eye movement) sleep. During that time, your eyes are literally moving rapidly, so if you're having a lot of vivid dreams, you may not be getting enough deep, restful sleep. In rare instances, consistent and frequent vivid dreams can indicate diabetes or even bipolar disorder, so if you are concerned about too-frequent vivid dreaming, check in with your doc to be on the safe side.

My husband snores like crazy. Does that mean he's sleeping well? Do you have any preferred solutions for his snoring, because now I can't sleep if he's sleeping in the room.

Nope, snoring doesn't mean he's sleeping well. People tend to snore for a few common reasons: their bodies are overtired, they've consumed too much alcohol or food too close to bedtime, they're overweight, or they're eating foods such as dairy products, which can produce mucus and inflammation in the upper airway. Cleaning out the dairy, cutting out the carbs, and engaging in regular exercise will do wonders for many people who snore. If your hubby's breathing starts and stops throughout the night, he should see a sleep specialist to look into sleep apnea. It's a treatable condition, but if left untreated, it can lead to heart and blood pressure issues.

Also, ladies, if your man isn't willing to try to stop snoring, get yourself a room of your own. You need your beauty sleep.

What's the Best Sleep Position?

I have seen patients with deep wrinkles in certain areas of their faces. When I ask them what position they sleep in, the sleep position often correlates with their wrinkles. Sleeping in the same position creates "sleeping lines," which eventually can become wrinkles. Also, if you favor one side in sleep, it will increase your chances of kidney stones on that side. How to fight this? Change positions, preferably sleeping on your back. If you have trouble sleeping on your back at first, place a wedge or massage roll under your knees, to keep you from rolling over during the night and to ease pressure on your lower back.

Nighty-Night

....

Countless conditions and events can disrupt sleep patterns—from work pressures to being wound up about an exciting event; from jet lag to turning back the clocks. So arm yourself with as many insomnia fighters as you can. And remember: although you might like change and variety in some aspects of your life, when it comes to sleep, your body doesn't! If your body could talk, it would tell you, "I want eight hours and I want them to start and end at the same time every day. You give me that, and I'll reward you with energy, consistent moods, better-looking skin, and generally good behavior."

Chapter 2

FOOD AND DIGESTION

The food you eat can be either
the safest and most powerful form of medicine
or the slowest form of poison.

—ANN WIGMORE, AUTHOR AND WHOLE FOODS ADVOCATE

We in naturopathic medicine have a saying: "If you don't know what to treat, start with the digestive tract." That is, when a doctor is perplexed and doesn't know what to do, she won't do harm, and may bring some healing, if she starts by helping her patient digest better. And there is excellent science to bear this out.

Digestive health is the key to lowering inflammation in the body, which drives all sorts of disease. Digestion is the key to absorption of the nutrients from the food we eat, an aid to weight loss, and the main method to detoxify the body (see chapter 5, "Detox-ification"), and the digestive tract is where your brain neurotransmitters are made—so it is a key to good mood, too.

To begin our gastroenterological discussion, it is first important to talk not about what you're eating, but *how* you're eating. That's right: *how*. Then we will spend time talking about what is best to eat to make you your most fabulous self.

How to Eat Mindfully

Have you ever been accused of "inhaling" your food? And what about that awful, and even painful, clogged sensation you feel when you're swallowing big bites, one right after another? This kind of eating feels bad because it *is* bad! Many of my patients experience a lot of burping and stomach pain, and often this is because of *how* they're eating. So I remind them to eat mind-fully and slowly, which reduces this pain by limiting the air they swallow. Michio Kushi, founder of the macro-biotic diet, is known to have said that if you chew any-thing one hundred times, it will be healthy. Let's be honest: chewing one hundred times won't turn a Big Mac into a Fuji apple. Yet Kushi does bring up a valid point: if you take a breath before each bite and chew small bites thoroughly, your food will digest better.

Eating mindfully means to be aware that you are

eating: It means taking in the aroma of the food, enjoying a reasonable bite, and chewing well (as opposed to swallowing large amounts whole). It means that you are ready to slow things down and allow healthy digestion to take place. Mindful eating is being appreciative that this food will nourish your body and give you life. Mindful eating ensures better digestion, and better digestion increases nutrient absorption, lowers inflammation, and creates a healthier you.

What Is Inflammation? Should I Change My Diet to Prevent It?

Inflammation is the tendency of your immune system to stay in attack and firefight mode. Eating quickly will keep your food from breaking down properly, and this will cause inflammation. Most of your immune system resides in your digestive tract. So, if you do not digest well, your immune system activates. Yes, some foods can really tick off your immune system: both foods that are cooked at high temperature (such as fried stuff) and things such as junk food. The so-called Mediterranean diet might be the least inflammatory diet of all, and it highlights lots of vegetables, healthy oils, beans, and raw nuts and seeds.

The Big Deal About Chewing

A lot of the latest nutrition news items (and big-name diets) focus on limiting your food intake—whether it is gluten-free, paleo, or what have you, many of these diets require avoiding carbohydrates in some way. While this might be a helpful approach for some individuals, it is important to back up a step to think about how we digest our food. When you take in food, your teeth grind it to bits in a mechanical process designed to increase the surface area of the food particles. This gives the digestive enzymes carried in your saliva the best chance to do their job of breaking down the food. Those carb-busting enzymes don't stand nearly as good a chance in a match against a large, thick hunk of poorly chewed food. The amylase enzyme in your saliva converts the shredded food starches to a form called maltose, which allows better digestion farther down your tract in your intestines. If this doesn't occur properly in your mouth, digestion suffers.

The bottom line? If you're not chewing well, the poorly broken down carbs can, and often do, lead to bloating, reflux, bacterial overgrowth, extra yeast in the digestive tract, skin issues, and inflammation in your intestines.

Slow Eating and Weight Loss

If you are trying to lose weight, remember this: when you eat too quickly, your stomach doesn't have enough time to tell the brain that you're full, so you end up eating more than you need or even want. I've seen patients adjust how they eat and lose weight without even changing the foods they eat. Chew on that.

The Air Up There

Many patients come to me experiencing significant burping and stomach pain. Eating mindfully and slowly reduces this pain by limiting the air you swallow (a medical condition called aerophagia). The ways to fix burping are:

- Eat mindfully.
- Avoid coffee, alcohol, dairy products, and chocolate; these are the top offenders.
- Take digestive enzymes with hydrochloric acid (HCl). In most cases, burping occurs not only due to excess air, but also because the body doesn't produce enough stomach acid (often due to stress, which shuts down digestion). Start with 500 mg of HCl (usually one gelcap), taken just after the first bite of each meal. Some people may need two or three with each meal. If this amount of HCl seems too strong and you have an acidic feeling or taste in your mouth after

taking it, try a gentler enzyme first, one that does not contain HCl. If you are experiencing regular stomach pain and long-term reflux, it's a good idea to visit your friendly neighborhood gastroenterologist for a checkup.

Eating Your Way to Fabulous

We've spoken about how to eat. Now we will spend time discussing the big question: "What should I eat?"

When you take a sick dog to the clinic, the first thing any self-respecting veterinarian will ask is "What are you feeding this dog?" Yet when it comes to human health, modern medicine still gives pitifully little attention to a most important pillar of health: food. There's no question that what you put in your mouth, how well you age, and how good your skin looks are all closely related.

Antioxidant Warriors

Antioxidants protect our body from the ravages of our own fuel-burning process (metabolism), wear and tear, and undernourishment. They give our genetic information the material it needs to survive and prosper. They also sop up free radicals (molecules that beat up our cells and age us quickly) and renew our repair systems. Moreover, they help clean out and restore our cell batteries (mitochondria).

The presence of an antioxidant in a plant food typically gives the food a deep, beautiful color. Prunes, carrots, and black beans are some of my favorite high-antioxidant foods. I've compiled the following shopping lists based on the items' antioxidant content. Purchase some you might not be getting enough of.

Dr. Pina's Favorite Spice: Turmeric

Turmeric is an ancient spice that is now known to contain a component called curcumin, which has antioxidant power. Turmeric lowers inflammation, lifts mood, and even fights cancer. I can't think of anyone who wouldn't benefit from turmeric—you can keep it in a salt shaker on your table and add it to your food. I love it in my morning oatmeal with a teaspoon of ghee and a touch of maple syrup. You can even add it to bathwater to unclog pores and soothe aching joints and muscles.

Shopping List: Fruits

❑ blueberries and other dark berries
❑ goji berries
❑ grapes

- ❏ mangoes
- ❏ melons (cantaloupe, honeydew)
- ❏ papayas
- ❏ pineapples
- ❏ pomegranates
- ❏ prunes
- ❏ tomatoes (yes, technically, they're a fruit)
- ❏ watermelon

Shopping List: Vegetables

- ❏ avocados
- ❏ beets
- ❏ carrots
- ❏ dark leafy greens like spinach
- ❏ kale, dragon kale
- ❏ pumpkin
- ❏ purple cabbage
- ❏ red bell peppers
- ❏ seaweed
- ❏ sweet potatoes
- ❏ Swiss chard, rainbow chard

Shopping List: Protein

- ❏ beans (black beans, kidney beans, navy beans, etc.)
- ❏ pistachios

❑ salmon
❑ shrimp and shellfish
❑ sunflower seeds
❑ tahini
❑ walnuts

Protein Requirements

For a healthy adult, the minimum pro-
tein requirements per day are about 0.8 g for every
2.2 lbs. of body weight. So, to figure this out, let's
use an example. Say you're 120 lbs. Divide 120 by
2.2, which gives you 54.5. Now multiply that
number by 0.8, which gives you 43.6 g of protein—it's not really a whole lot. If you are an avid
exerciser (which is great), it means you need more
protein, so multiply by 1 g instead of 0.8. For elite
athletes (at the level of an Olympian or professional), multiply by 1.2 g. Here's the equation:

(weight in pounds / 2.2) x 0.8 g =

_____ grams of protein needed per day

The Essential Organics

All meats you consume should be antibiotic- and
hormone-free. According to the Environmental
Working Group (a nonprofit and noncommercial or-

ganization that is an excellent resource for environmental health), some produce contains more pesticides than others. The foods that contain the most pesticides are:

- apples
- celery
- cherry tomatoes
- collard greens
- cucumbers
- grapes
- kale
- nectarines
- peaches
- potatoes
- snap peas
- spinach
- strawberries
- sweet peppers

When consuming the foods on this list, always choose organic. For more about organic foods and products, check out www.EWG.org.

Organic: Price Versus Value

Organic foods are totally and completely worth the money. Don't believe anyone who says otherwise. Pesticides in foods are linked to early puberty in young girls, diabetes, leukemia, Parkinson's disease, and other illnesses. Also, when you use pesticides to protect a plant, the plant produces far fewer of the phytonutrients it uses for its own self-protection, which means less good nutrition for your body.

Frozen Versus Fresh

Both frozen and fresh are quite good. Fresh food has higher enzymes and antioxidant levels. More enzymes mean better digestibility, and more antioxidants mean more antiaging power. But frozen can be excellent, too. When frozen food is thawed, many nutrients can be "freed" as the cells of the fruit or vegetable burst open. Moreover, research shows that frozen blueberries deliver more phytonutrients than fresh ones.

Some people don't have easy access to fresh fruits and vegetables. If this applies to you, keeping produce in the freezer allows you to have it whenever you need it, and fruit and veggies are much better for you than a bag of chips. So freeze away for a rainy day!

Is Soy Good for Me?

This is an especially important question for women with a history of breast or uterine cancer.

✴ Soy is thought to contain phytoestrogens. This word literally means "plant estrogens," which is misleading to both doctors and the public alike, who assume that it acts like an estrogen hormone and will contribute to breast cancer. Studies out of Asia show that women who eat soy foods regularly have much lower rates of breast cancer than women in the United States, who eat little to no soy. One case-controlled study from 2008 looked at more than twenty-four thousand Japanese women and found that those with the highest soy isoflavone levels had the lowest cancer rates. A large meta-analysis (a study of many studies) published in 2015 also showed that soy food consumption lowered breast cancer risk in Chinese women. Breast cancer incidence is much lower in Asia than in Western countries, where isoflavone levels are about 0.5 percent of those in Asia. It also appears that after moving to the United States and eating our food, Asian women see their breast cancer rates switch to U.S. rates within one generation.

It is true that soy's isoflavones can act like weak estrogen molecules. But instead of acting to promote cancer, they appear to be protective. The weak "estrogens" in soy actually block the more aggressive, cancer-causing estrogens—as such, they lower the effect of those estrogens. This is also the effect of Tamoxifen, a drug that serves to prevent breast cancer recurrence: it decreases the effect of aggressive estrogens. Additionally, soy isoflavones help shut off genes that can cause cancer, by acting as methylators, molecules that lock up the genes so they are not expressed.

As with most foods, when soy is consumed in excessive amounts it can cause some imbalances. For instance, soy may inhibit thyroid function, lower mineral absorption, or even create an allergic response. Excessive soy consumption in young children may imbalance hormone levels. However, when eaten in reasonable amounts (about 8 or 10 g a day), soy protein is perfectly safe.

In our clinic, we highly recommend natural and fermented forms of soy, such as edamame, natto, miso, and tempeh. While some soy milk and tofu may not be harmful, these more processed sources of soy may increase sensitivity in some individuals. Also it is good to remember that soy is the food most likely to be genetically modified. So make sure your soy is non-GMO (genetically modified organism). Persons with blood type A seem to do fairly well with soy in the diet, while blood type O individuals seem to be more reactive. (See the section "The Blood Type Diet" on page 44 for a more detailed discussion of blood types and diet.)

Cauliflower and Other Superfoods

Any woman interested in protecting herself against breast cancer and balancing her hormones wants to eat foods from the genus *Brassica*. These include bok choy, broccoli, Brussels sprouts, and cauliflower. These foods contain indole-3-carbinol, which helps the liver process hormones and create healthy estrogen balances in your body to lower breast cancer risk and protect against bone thinning (osteoporosis). They also contain sulfur compounds that stop colon cancer from forming, lower inflammation, and keep the heart healthy.

My Two Favorite Diets

Patients ask me all the time, "Dr. Pina, if you had to pick one diet to live by, which one would it be?" I think food plans are best when tailored to the individual, but, all right, if I were being forced to answer, and if I didn't know you, I could feel comfortable telling you where to start: the Mediterranean diet and the blood type diet

The Mediterranean Diet

The Mediterranean diet hails from the land of my Sicilian parents and stretches to all shores touched by the Mediterranean Sea. In this land, the rich soil produces some of the most beautiful and healthiest farm-to-table foods, which benefit both the body and the mind. Numerous studies over the years have shown the benefits to the heart, blood vessels, and brain function of the Mediterranean diet.

One of my favorite places is Sardinia, an island off the coast of Italy and one of the most beautiful spots in the country—Italy untouched. Sardinia is one of the areas in the world called blue zones, where many people live healthily above one hundred years. A main factor for this longevity? It's the food.

Can the Mediterranean Diet Prevent Alzheimer's Disease?

Alzheimer's disease is the sixth leading cause of death in the United States, and we women make up almost two-thirds of the disease's victims. According to the Alzheimer's Association, as of this writing Alzheimer's is the only disease that cannot be prevented or slowed. (It sounds to me like they haven't been reading about the Mediterranean diet.) Researchers from Johns Hopkins teamed up with the University of London and pored through stacks of medical literature to see what was available to prevent this dreaded disease. Published in April 2015 in *The American Journal of Psychiatry*, the research shows that people with mild memory issues earlier in life (a predictor of Alzheimer's) who switched to the Mediterranean diet had a much lower likelihood of getting the disease. The researchers also found that low folate levels and high blood sugar were linked to the development of Alzheimer's. Folate is naturally found in green leafy vegetables. (The word *folate* comes from the Latin *folium*, which means "leaf.") So eat your greens!

Common Factors for Longevity in Blue Zones

The world's blue zones are where people tend to have the greatest health and longevity. These areas are: Sardinia, in Italy; Loma Linda, California; Okinawa, Japan; and Nicoya Peninsula, Costa Rica. Contrary to previous thought, main factors are not based on genetics but instead are diet- and lifestyle-based. These factors are:

- engaging in daily movement;
- living with a sense of purpose;
- consuming a diet rich in beans, absent of sugar and white flour, and containing minimal meat; and
- enjoying a strong social community.

Here are some pointers to get you started following the Mediterranean diet:

Lots

- **Green vegetables.** These are hard to overdose on. Shoot for at least one to two cups a day.
- **Fruits.** Try to eat organic fruits with the skin on (one to two cups a day).
- **Healthy monounsaturated fats.** You can supplement with fish oil (one teaspoon a day), olive oil (one teaspoon a day), and a tablespoon of flax meal added to your foods. Also try to limit saturated fats, such as red meat and butter. A little butter (e.g., one teaspoon a day) is okay; a lot is not.
- **Legumes (beans).** Most of us do not eat enough beans. If you are eating beans for the first time, go slow. The gas can creep up on you while your intestinal bacteria get used to the extra fiber. Aim for half a cup to one cup a day.
- **Fish.** Specifically low-mercury fish such as wild salmon, sardines, trout, whitefish, flounder, and tilapia. Fish three times a week is wonderful.

In Moderation

- **Whole grains.** Eat whole-grain cereals and hearty, unrefined breads. I like Fitness Bread and sprouted breads from Ezekiel. If you are gluten-sensitive, limit yourself to gluten-free grains such as quinoa, gluten-free oatmeal, millet, and pure buckwheat (despite the name, buckwheat does not have wheat in it).
- **Nuts.** Take in a half cup of raw nuts every day. Raw is healthier than roasted, for the oils are best unheated.

In Small Amounts

- **Milk and dairy products.** Keep these to a minimum. If you are sensitive to cow's milk, skip them altogether.
- **Meat and meat products.** Minimize your intake of these, and when you do eat meat, look for grass-fed, organic, hormone- and antibiotic-free versions.
- **Alcohol.** Keep your intake moderate. (See the box "How Much Alcohol Is Safe?")

When you're ready to get cookin' on a food plan based on the Mediterranean diet, please visit www

.DrPinaND.com/Mediterranean to get some of my fabulous recipes.

How Much Alcohol Is Safe?

While there may be some benefit from red wine, such as in preventing diabetes and helping heart health, in 1988 the International Agency for Research on Cancer declared alcohol a carcinogen, which means it causes cancer. Today, alcohol is probably responsible for 6 percent of all cancers, and most of the increased cancer incidence over the years is due to the fact that women are drinking more. It seems women are more sensitive to the cancer effects than men, and breast cancer seems to be the most concerning. Most experts are hesitant to recommend any amount of wine as safe, but general guidelines suggest no more than one drink a day for women and two drinks for men. For people with known cancer risk, it may be best to avoid alcohol altogether, or to save it only for special occasions.

Love Your EVOO (Extra-Virgin Olive Oil)

One of the most vital foods in the Mediterranean diet is olive oil, particularly the extra-virgin kind (TV chef

Rachael Ray's famous "E-V-O-O"). This precious liquid gold contains monounsaturated fats and phenol compounds—which are similar to alcohol molecules, but these don't get you drunk. These fats and phenols can influence more than one hundred genes that control the aging process. Olive oil also protects against osteoporosis and Alzheimer's. Armed with omega-9 oleic acids not easily found in other foods, olive oil is a potent foe of breast cancer.

A 2013 study found that extra-virgin olive oil has greater benefits than regular olive oil. (I'm a bit of an olive oil enthusiast, so bear with me on this one.) I strongly recommend you don't go cheap here. Purchase organic (so there'll be no toxic compounds), cold-pressed, extra-virgin olive oil. The "extra" part means the oil is simply pressed, without chemicals. And it typically comes from young olives, which yield higher-quality oil. Buy it in small glass bottles that you can keep in a dark, cool place. Larger containers mean the oil will be more exposed to air and will oxidize, which makes a healthy oil not so healthy anymore. Also, don't cook olive oil at high temperatures—it's made for lightly cooking and sautéing. If your recipe calls for a hotter flame, there are other choices: coconut oil, avocado oil, high-heat safflower oil, and peanut oil.

❊ Research on the Mediterranean Diet

How does the Mediterranean diet help? Over the past decade, research about this food plan has been booming. From it, we are learning that the diet lowers inflammation, blood sugar, and bad cholesterol and increases repair factors in the brain. A 2015 paper in the journal *Endocrine, Metabolic, and Immune Disorders—Drug Targets* (not the catchiest name for a journal) showed that when people were on the Mediterranean diet, they had substantially lower levels of C-reactive protein (a marker for inflammation), much better blood sugar levels, and even lower blood pressure. Papers from a Spanish group of researchers who originally studied these foods showed the clear ability of this diet to reduce anxiety and depression. And in 2015, *The Journal of the American Medical Association* showed that cancers, including breast cancer, can be staved off by eating a Mediterranean diet. Researchers have found that olive oil components suppressed the breast cancer–promoting gene HER2 by encouraging early cancer cells to commit hara-kiri—that is, kill themselves voluntarily. Very recent research from *JAMA Internal Medicine* looked at seventy-five hundred women over a five-year period and showed that breast cancer risk was cut 62 percent in women who ingested high amounts of olive oil. These results are impressive, for these women had type 2 diabetes, which made them even more likely to get cancer.

The Blood Type Diet

Patients who have a lot of inflammation in their bodies present in my office with things such as rashes, hives, eczema, or internal problems such as autoimmune disease, blood vessel disease, or even cancer. I look to support them with a diet more specific to their sensitivities. Strategies such as an elimination diet and blood testing are fine, but I've found that the blood type diet offers the quickest results.

✳ Your blood type gives medical professionals clues as to how your immune system might react to certain foods, showing us what system of proteins resides on your cell membranes. These proteins can interact either favorably or unfavorably with proteins in your food. When the reaction is unfavorable, inflammation is the result.

Written by Dr. Peter D'Adamo, *Eat Right for Your Type* has been an effective guide for me when advising patients what foods may work best for them. While no diet book is 100 percent accurate for every person, this one will likely hit closer to the mark. In my practice, I have found it to be more accurate than food allergy testing.

For example, the general tenets for blood type A (my type) are to eat plenty of fish, pineapple, and pumpkin seeds, and to avoid dairy and red meat. Blood type O people do best with grass-fed red meats, but need to stay away from all gluten. Blood type B people will react negatively to chicken, but do fine with most cheese. And those with the AB blood type do especially well with lamb and yogurt, but may need to minimize shellfish. No matter your blood type, though, plants and green vegetables still prove most beneficial.

Should I Follow the Caveman/ Paleo Diet?

Two hundred thousand years ago, we humans generally ate very little and had very physical lives in order to survive. We ate berries, nuts, and an occasional killed animal, and probably burned as many calories just to get that food. And we released a lot of stress hormones in the process.

Today's woman might stand in line for a doughnut and coffee at Dunkin' Donuts and scarf down more calories in a rushed five minutes at her desk than she would be able to burn in an entire day. In the world of diners, dives, and drive-ins, we're surrounded by far more food than we need.

The Paleo program includes eating fewer carbs and moving a lot. That makes sense. This behavior fixes diabetes and inflammatory disease like a charm. While my patients think the diet is magic, it's really just physiology.

Some patients, however, don't do so well eating all that meat, and grilling can be unhealthy due to the production of AGEs. (We will discuss these in the section "Turn Down the Heat and Limit Your AGEs" on page 54.) Also, I find too many people who go Paleo don't focus on eating green vegetables and end up restricting beans and healthy grains such as quinoa. While restriction may be right for some people in the short term, a strict Paleo plan tends to fall flat in the long term.

How do you know if meat is right for you? Look at your blood type. Type O people tend to do great with meat, while blood type As do better with vegetarian meals and fish. If you are blood type B, most meats are okay (except for chicken), and ABs can generally have a little of everything.

How many calories do I burn by standing in line at Dunkin' Donuts for one hour?
50

How many calories in an average doughnut?
289

Whole Versus Fat-Free Milk

Many patients tell me they drink skim milk for better health. I will tell you now: skim is not better for you. You may not know this, but because the natural fat has been removed from skim milk, powdered milk is mixed into it to thicken it and make it more appealing. Powdered milk is a known contributor to inflammation, and an artery clogger. Also, many vitamins are stripped away along with the fat. Studies from Harvard have shown that low-fat milk is associated with gaining weight, while whole-fat milk is not. Generally, I do not recommend milk to patients, as it is an inflammatory food. But if you must drink it, go full fat!

Butter Versus Ghee

Ghee is basically butter that's been heated and put through a sieve to remove the creamy top layer, which contains all the dairy proteins. So if you are lactose intolerant (sensitive to dairy), ghee is great. Both ghee and butter contain butyrate (from *butyrum*, the Latin word for butter), a molecule that helps keep the intestines super healthy. Both butter and ghee in moderate quantities (from one teaspoon up to one tablespoon a day) are great. But if you are sensitive to dairy, go for the ghee. It's delicious.

Eggs

Eggs are eggs-cellent! (Forgive me.) Years ago, we vilified the egg for its cholesterol—until we realized that it's actually simple carbs and sugar that clog our blood vessels. Eggs are an excellent source of protein (about 8 g per egg). They have carotenes (which give their yolks a beautiful yellow color) and a few hard-to-find nutrients such as choline, which boosts memory; and lutein, which protects our eyes from aging. The yolk of the egg helps create younger skin and lusher hair, from its nutrients biotin and zinc. The healthiest way to eat an egg is poached or boiled (hard or soft)—this way the yolk isn't broken. When the yolk is broken, the cholesterol in it oxidizes, making it less healthful. And eggs are not dairy—they just sit next to the milk at the supermarket.

Vegetable Protein

Think you absolutely *have* to obtain most of your protein from animals? Think again. There are plenty of ways to get enough protein from vegetables. Tofu has about 12 g of protein per 3 oz, while quinoa has 8 g per cup. Greek yogurt has 23 g per half cup; lentils have about 9 g and Great Northern beans 7.5 g per half cup. Tempeh is the king of vegetarian protein, with more than 20 g per half cup. A delicious way to add protein to your vegetarian meal is to spread almond butter on a celery stick. Or try pumpkin and sunflower seeds on top of your salad, and throw a heaping scoop of natural vanilla-flavored rice protein into your favorite smoothie.

Eating Well by Cleaning out the Junk

I have been dairy-free for several years, and I started because I felt it was going to reduce my allergies, which it did, and help me lose weight, which it did.

—FRAN DRESCHER, ACTRESS

Okay, it's time to cut the crap. This is the part of the book where I sound like a nag and say, "Don't eat this" and "Don't eat that." If you want healthy skin, and greater energy and glow, then you may want to limit your relationship with the following tempting foods:

- Simple carbohydrates: bread, pasta, bagels, gluten, white rice;
- Sugary foods: juice, cookies, cake, pie, ice cream, candy;

- Dairy products: cheese, cow's milk, cream, ice cream; and
- Artificial junk: dyes (including tartrazine and F, D, and C colors) and any word you don't recognize in an ingredient list.

Patients are always telling me that after cutting out items from this list, they feel better than ever. I hear comments like:

- "My skin cleared up."
- "The colors of the day are more vibrant."
- "I don't bloat and swell."
- "I can see my muscles without exercising more."
- "I see better."
- "My energy has shot up."
- "I can poop!"

Remember, this isn't a fast. If you don't know what to eat, go back to the beginning of the chapter, where I talk about all the beautiful, healthy foods you can indulge in. You should eat as much as you want— just keep it healthy most of the time.

So, the Occasional Treat Is Okay?

As of this writing, my daughter, Sophia, is seven years old. My husband and I tell her that it is okay to eat fun things such as dessert as an occasional treat, but not as everyday foods. If you are a puritan and *never* indulge, that's no fun, and that strategy pretty much never works. Instead, by having an occasional treat you'll never feel deprived, and will therefore be much less likely to binge or cheat. Maybe have "Pizza Sunday" or "Friday night fries," enjoying your favorite indulgence in a reasonable amount once a week. When I have pizza, I also eat plenty of greens, so even this cheat food is an opportunity to consume vegetables.

Gluten-Free: Fad or Something to Take Seriously?

Gluten-free is pretty much the new black. Everywhere you go, there are gluten-free options. Is this a just fad, or good medicine?

Many people would benefit from avoiding gluten. This protein is eaten by most people every day, if not a few times a day. Any strong protein the immune system sees coming through the digestive tract is, after a while, likely to start creating inflammation. Since we eat a lot of gluten, many of us become sensitive, and this sets off reactions. I see this with people who eat a lot of soy—after a while, the system starts to react to the soy protein. So, what's the best approach? If you think you are sensitive to gluten, lay off it for three months. Then add it back in—but not every day. Rotate it in every few days, and look for other healthy foods to replace it.

Glycemic Index and Load

Many people avoid carbs to lose weight. Yet not all carbs are created equal in the fight against fat. The glycemic index and glycemic load are rankings that describe how big a sugar hit a given food is going to have in your body. Carbs that have a higher glycemic index and load do not contain much fiber and will break down into a lot of sugar quickly. Low-glycemic carbs break down into a little sugar and have lots of fiber to keep the stomach satisfied. When the sugar hit is high, your body responds by producing more insulin, which automatically tells your body to pack fat cells and create inflammation. Inflammation pushes the heart disease and cancer buttons in your body. From a glycemic standpoint, the best carbs are vegetables, oatmeal, and fruits such as berries. The worst carbs are alcohol, fruit juice, bagels, doughnuts, and white bread.

Turn Down the Heat and Limit Your AGEs

Pretty strong research is mounting that tells us it isn't just *what* you eat or don't eat that's important. Now we are learning that *how food is cooked* also impacts your glow—big time. Want to dim your glow and keep your skin looking unhealthy? Eat barbecue and fried foods such as doughnuts and chips every day. It will show up on your skin in the form of rashes, eczema, age spots, and wrinkles.

✳ What makes these foods so nasty? It's the heat they're cooked in. When proteins and sugar crystals get together at a nice high temperature (let's say in a frying pan or high-heat oven, on the grill, or at 98.6 degrees in your body), they start to "glycate," meaning the protein and the sugar stick together and heat up. In the heat of this moment, damage is done to proteins. This process takes place both in the frying pan and in your body. In your body this damage will advance the look of aging by breaking down your skin's keratin and collagen, as well as speed the clock in your vessels, organs, nerves, and all your tissues.

Heating foods at high temperatures results in advanced glycation end products (known as AGEs), a significant factor in skin and body aging. The acronym AGE is perfect, for AGEs do just that—they age you. The more sugar involved, the more glycation takes place, which is another reason to cut down on both sugar and simple carbs.

These AGEs then bind to your immune system, on receptors appropriately called receptors for advanced glycation end products. The acronym for this one? RAGE. Guess what happens when the AGEs dock on to the RAGEs. Jeffrey Bland, a nutritional biochemist, explains how these interactions cause our bodies (especially the fat cells) to become angry and inflamed, leaving us with an "enRAGEd" system, and an inability to burn fat. This inflammation causes not only your tissues to break down but also the oils and fats in your blood to go rancid. This process is called oxidation and is one of the reasons eating foods with antioxidants is so important for good health. AGEs are not good for your glow or your cardiovascular system.

One Little Chip

A Polish study conducted in 2009 on the cute little potato chip revealed that regularly eating these for four weeks increased both the oxidation of bad cholesterol (LDL) and levels of C-reactive protein (CRP). Oxidation of LDL will drive atherosclerosis, the clogging of your blood vessels. CRP is a marker for inflammation in the body that increases when the cardiovascular system is at risk. High CRP is also linked to anxiety, depression, fatigue, and just plain looking and feeling old before your time. So all of a sudden, that cute little chip isn't so cute anymore.

To avoid the ravages of AGEs, focus on foods that are cooked at lower temperatures. Doing more boiling, poaching, and stewing and less frying, broiling, and roasting can decrease daily AGE intake by up to 50 percent. Weight your diet toward foods such as soups, slow-cooker dishes, boiled foods, low-temperature baked items, and lightly sautéed dishes.

Look at the AGE kilounit differences for a three-ounce piece of chicken:

Oven-fried	9,000
Deep fried	6,700
Broiled	5,250
Roasted	4,300
Boiled	1,000

The typical recommended daily AGE content is about 16,000 kilounits. So, just eating a little fried chicken can put you way over the top, and age you fast.

Microwaves

I'm not a fan of the microwave, but it does seem that food cooked in one has an AGE content not much different from that of boiled food. Microwaves do, however, increase the oxidation in fatty foods, and will chemically change the forms of the proteins in your food. We don't know for sure if this has an unhealthy cumulative effect in your body by causing subtle damage to your system. My advice is to use microwaves sparingly.

Grill, Baby, Grill?

While I love chef Bobby Flay as much as anyone, many patients have come to me after watching some Paleo health program on TV that says grilled meats are the way to go. Yet these programs never take AGEs into account, and leave my patients wondering why they are feeling worse after eating this way!

Are Raw Foods the Best?

The AGE level in raw foods is near zero. The problem, however, is that most people cannot sustain themselves on raw foods exclusively. While nutritionally great in theory, raw foods are really hard for the body to break down. In Chinese medicine, these are considered very "cold" energetically (as opposed to temperature-wise) and will "douse your digestive fire." Before I learned how to eat healthy, I had a strong personal history of irritable bowel syndrome, and I know that eating too many raw foods will make it worse. Some salads, greens juices, and raw veggies and fruit are fine if your digestive system is healthy. But when it's struggling, raw can be too hard to handle, and can limit the absorption of nutrients.

Healthy Weight

I have to work really hard. I have a voluptuous body.
I am not one of those skinny girls.
I like to enjoy life.

—DOUTZEN KROES, ACTRESS
AND FORMER VICTORIA'S SECRET MODEL

For this section, I want to talk about how to lose weight. Before I do, though, I want you to remember you are beautiful the way you are. Moreover, there is something called the obesity paradox: research from the Mayo Clinic suggests that people who are slightly overweight may actually live longer than people who are underweight. So my thought is that it is okay to have a few more pounds than the skinny models in the magazines. However, if you are significantly over-weight and are at high risk for diabetes, cardiovascular disease, and cancer, or if you feel your current weight is not right for you, then losing weight can be helpful.

"I Eat So Little, and I Still Can't Lose a Pound"

This is possibly the most common complaint I hear in my practice, especially from patients in their forties and beyond. Yet now I am seeing more and more teens and twentysomethings with the same concern. The fact is, if you are trying to eat fewer calories to lose weight and it's not working, it may not be about food. I am going to tell you what simple things you need to do first. This plan works—and it doesn't even change anything you eat!

Weight Loss Step 1: Get Enough Sleep

Lack of sleep is proven to do three things:

- It messes up your blood sugar, which makes you crave sweets.

🍃 It slows your metabolism, which means you
  don't burn fat as efficiently.

🍃 It makes your body deposit more fat in the
  places you don't want it.

Sleep is so important that it's the very first step toward healthy beauty covered in this book. If you need
to, reread chapter 1, "Your Beauty Sleep," and make
sure you get your eight hours.

Weight Loss Step 2: Work on the Stress

There's an old saying: "It's not what you're eating, it's
what's eating you."

Yes ma'am. Stress is a big problem. When stress
hormones (cortisol and adrenaline) are high, your
body holds on to fat. Why? Because in the wild,
stressed animals are usually stressed because there's not
enough food, so when you are stressed, your primitive
brain (located in the bump above the back of your
neck) sends out hunger signals. Whether it's because
the boss is yelling at you or your partner is being a
jerk, your natural stress response makes you want to
eat more calories, and you will also burn fewer calories and fat. Lack of sleep also increases stress hormones, making it a double whammy.

Create a meditation and relaxation schedule that
you follow every day, without fail. Just five minutes
twice a day is great. If you have a lot of stressful and

negative thoughts and you need some relaxation, you can work on this in chapter 4.

Weight Loss Step 3: Exercise

Not a big surprise. Exercise will help you burn the fat, sleep better, and metabolize stress hormones so they don't make you feel so stressed. Not bad! Oh, and you'll look leaner, too.

Exercise a minimum of four times a week for a half hour. (The next chapter will get you moving.)

Weight Loss Step 4: Have Sex

Like exercise, sex burns stress hormones, which helps you sleep better and reduces food cravings. Sex helps your body make oxytocin, which is the hormone of love and facilitates bonding with other people. Women also have a better body image when having sex regularly. Sexual activity burns about ninety calories a half hour—much better than watching a movie.

What about self-serving? Yes, masturbation can achieve some of the benefits of partner-driven sexual activity, including our improved sense of self-esteem and relaxation. Like sex and anything else, if you are overdoing it or using it to avoid connection with others, then that may be something to work on with a therapist. In general, if you don't have a partner—go for it. If you do have a partner, he or she can help!

Either way, try to enjoy regular sexual activity a few times a week.

What's Oxytocin, and How Do I Get Some?

Oxytocin is an important feel-good neuro-transmitter. People who typically feel lonely have lower levels of oxytocin.

To increase your oxytocin:

- Get a massage.
- Hug someone.
- Relax and eat a nice meal with friends.
- Supplement with lithium orotate (it's not a drug, but a mineral similar to potassium).
- Get busy (aka physical intimacy—that's code for sex).
- Engage in physical activity and exercise.
- Become involved in your community.

Weight Loss Step 5: Enjoy Your Food!

As we discussed earlier in this chapter, eating mindfully is key. The slower you eat, the more time your stomach has to tell your brain you're getting enough calories. Scarfing down your food lets you sneak by hundreds of extra calories before your brain tells you to stop. Go slow, and you will naturally eat a lot less.

Whatever you eat, enjoy it as much as you can. Eat it S-L-O-W-L-Y, and savor every bite.

Weight Loss Step 6: Practice Intermittent Fasting

With intermittent fasting, you eat only during a ten-hour period. This helps your body by letting your digestive tract and liver take a break and it brings your body into a state that allows it to burn off the fat more easily. Studies show that even if you do not curb your food intake or change a calorie, if you intermittently fast like this, you will lose weight.

I recommend you start eating at 8:00 a.m. and then do not eat past 6:00 p.m. If your lifestyle requires a different schedule (say, eating between 10:00 a.m. and 8:00 p.m.), that is fine, too—just try not to eat too much food too close to bedtime, for it may interrupt your sleep.

During this ten-hour period of eating, you can have three meals and one or two snacks. This will allow you to go fourteen hours without food. (Don't worry; it's not that bad—eight hours of this time you will spend sleeping.)

Weight Loss Step 7: Get Your Blood Tested

To work on weight loss properly, sometimes we need to check under the hood. Every patient I see for weight loss gets the following tests:

- **Iron panel with ferritin.** Iron and ferritin (a protein that handles iron storage) are important. When you have low iron and don't store enough of it, your body shuts down its

metabolism to save energy. That means slow
fat loss.

- **Full thyroid panel with antibodies.** Healthy
thyroid function helps keep you firing on all
cylinders. We check your antibodies to see if
your immune system might be slowing your
thyroid function. If your thyroid is sluggish:

    Exercise in the cold (if it's summer, take up
    swimming in a cool pool). Cold kicks up
    thyroid function.

    Eat seaweed. Its micronutrients are great for
    thyroid function.

  If your antibodies are high:

    Take selenium. Two hundred micrograms (mcg,
    which is one-thousandth of a milligram) a day
    helps lower inflammation of the thyroid.

    Clean out the gluten. I have seen a number of
    patients dump their thyroid hormone
    prescription just by getting rid of this
    inflammatory food.

    Follow the Mediterranean diet more closely. It is a
    great anti-inflammatory plan.

- **Hemoglobin A1c.** This test looks at blood
sugar levels over a three-month period. If your
level is higher than 5.3 percent, get serious
about limiting sugar and simple carbs such as
the "white foods": bread, cake, cookies, pasta,
gluten, white rice, and bagels.

- **Leptin.** This hormone is an important control

for weight loss. It can regulate thyroid function and fertility, too. If leptin is high, return it to normal by getting serious about cutting all carbohydrates for three months, including fruits and beans. While I don't like removing these healthy foods, after the three months your body should reset itself, and then the beans and fruit can be added back to your diet. I have my patients do a detox (see chapter 5, "Detoxification"), since environmental chemicals will stop the body from losing fat and will keep leptin levels high.

Testosterone. This hormone is not just for men. Women make it, too, and need it to maintain sexual drive, to build muscle, and to lose weight. Have your free and total testosterone checked. If either level is low, don't start taking hormones. Instead:

Get enough sleep.

Exercise.

Have sex.

Eat plenty of protein, at least 50 g a day.

Take ginseng. It stimulates the hypothalamus (in the middle of the brain) to make testosterone naturally and helps the body adapt to stress.

Take tongkat ali (200 mg a day) to raise testosterone naturally.

Tongkat Ali? What's That?

Eurycoma longifolia (tongkat ali) is a Southeast Asian plant long known to help improve overall quality of life. Researchers in a 2013 *Journal of the International Society of Sports Nutrition* study gave either 200 mg of tongkat ali or sugar pills to sixty-four volunteers. Those who received the herb for four weeks showed lower stress hormones, lifted emotions, and increased testosterone by an average of 37 percent.

Weight Loss Step 8: Supplement Your Serotonin and Curb Cravings with Chromium

As much as the media love the word *miracle*, there's no miracle weight loss supplement. Having said that, I will admit that I do love two: 5-HTP and chromium.

✐ **5-HTP (5-hydroxytryptophan)** is a version of tryptophan that has been proven to help overweight women reduce their appetites and eat less. Tryptophan supports your brain's natural serotonin levels. (Serotonin is a neurotransmitter that helps keep mood positive and plays a role in appetite.) Start with 50 mg of 5-HTP twice a day in between meals, but take it with a little carbohydrate, such as a handful of blueberries. This supplement is also effective for anxiety and depression—so, it's great if you have a poor mood and need to lose weight, too!

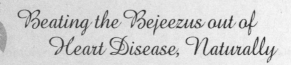 **Chromium**, a mineral that helps balance blood sugar, is found naturally in tomatoes, brewer's yeast, and onions. While chromium alone will not melt fat, when combined with a healthful diet and exercise, it will help calm cravings and support healthy body weight. Try 200 mcg three times a day with meals.

Beating the Bejeezus out of Heart Disease, Naturally

A 2014 study published in the *Journal of the American College of Cardiology* looked at almost twenty-one thousand men* and found that the 1 percent who ate well, exercised, stayed trim, and did not consume too much alcohol reduced their chance of a heart problem by at least 80 percent.

Wow—no drug does that!

* Hey, ever notice that a lot of research is on men? Why is that? It's because women have more hormonal fluctuations that can confuse researchers, so the researchers focus on men to make their studies easier. Please write to our government to tell my old employer the National Institutes of Health to start more protocols to study women's health!

Counting Calories

You'll notice I haven't recommended that you start counting every calorie. I find that this doesn't work well. (Actually, it doesn't work at all.) What seems to work is to choose whole foods that are nutrient dense and filling (vegetables, fruits, beans, fish, lean organic and grass-fed meats), and save the cakes, cookies, breads, and bagels for rare (enjoyable) occasions. (I'm a Sicilian girl, so I still eat the occasional pasta and pizza dish. But now I eat slowly and enjoy the process—and I don't overdo it.) Vegetables and plenty of fiber fill the stomach and signal to the pressure receptors that we've eaten enough. Nutrient-poor foods such as baloney sandwiches and ice cream don't have that effect.

"Can I Use Artificial Sweeteners to Lose Weight?"

The verdict is in: diet sodas and artificial sweeteners (such as aspartame, sucralose, and saccharine) are now known to cause as many heart problems as sugar, and they are toxic to your brain! Almost any ingredient with -ol at the end of its name (e.g., mannitol and sorbitol) is a sugar alcohol, and those are molecules your digestive system can't handle. (The exception is xylitol, which can be good for sinus issues.)

My favorite natural sweetener is stevia. Stevia is three hundred times sweeter than sugar (so use it lightly), and it may actually help balance blood sugar.

In general, though, I advise patients to reduce any sweetener use, and to get accustomed to recognizing and enjoying the *real* taste of food without added sweeteners. The naturally bitter taste of food actually triggers healthy stomach responses, turning on healthy digestion.

Chapter 3

MOVE IN YOUR
GLOW ZONE

Get comfortable being uncomfortable.

———

—JILLIAN MICHAELS,
PERSONAL TRAINER AND REALITY TV STAR

So, how to move farther into your glow zone?
You've got to move it!

From a medical standpoint, exercise is one of the
top drugs for amazing health, boasting phenomenal
efficacy with few side effects. Numerous studies have
powerfully shown that it doesn't take a whole lot of
exercise to decrease the risk of death, prevent the development of cancer, lower the risk of osteoporosis,
and increase life expectancy. Then, of course, there
are the added benefits of exercise: feeling and looking
fabulous. There's no drug in the world that can deliver

this, and no drug ever will. When you exercise your muscles, you break down skeletal tissue, which calls upon the body's immune system and restorative capacity to regenerate and renew. If you exercise too hard, however, you overwhelm the system and break more than it can handle, and you get hurt. So balance is the key.

A 2015 study out of Copenhagen followed almost two thousand joggers and sixteen thousand nonjoggers for up to thirty-five years and found that male runners lived 6.2 years longer and the women runners 5.6 years longer than people who did not run. There's no drug that does this. Imagine if there were. It would be the billion-dollar blockbuster of the century.

Work Harder or Smarter?

....

You can be an overachiever, but it's going to work against you. You'll be happy to know that in the just-mentioned Copenhagen study, the greatest benefits for living longer were found in the group that did the least amount of work! In that study, the "I can do better than you" types ran a faster pace of seven or more miles per hour and ran four or more hours a week. It turned out that not only did they not live longer, but they lost most or all the longevity benefits and had the same life expectancy as people who did nothing. The light and moderate joggers had the greatest life expectancy—they ran between only 1.0 and 2.5 hours weekly at five to seven miles an hour. Sometimes less really is more.

Along these same lines, a small 2008 Swiss study (sixty-nine subjects) presented at a European Society of Cardiology meeting showed that previously sedentary people who switched from riding escalators and elevators to taking the stairs for twelve weeks changed markers in their blood that suggested they would cut their risk of dying prematurely by 15 percent. In that relatively short period, these people reduced their body fat, trimmed their waistlines, and lowered their blood pressure. Not bad for taking the steps.

Exercise Makes You Look Better

Okay, so forget about the fantastic health benefits for a minute. Exercise will make you look good. *Really* good.

According to an April 2014 article in the *New York Times*, exercise not only appears to help your skin look younger, but it can also reverse the aging process, even if you start exercising later in life. Add to that the aesthetic benefits of being firmer, having better muscle tone and posture, and fitting into smaller clothes. Also you can't put a value on feeling strong. It's empowering and it simply makes you move differently, with more confidence. Being fit is sexy, and that's never going to change.

✳ One of the main causes of older-looking skin is something unrelated to sun damage: it's the stiffening of our skin. As we age, the outer skin layer (the epidermis) gets drier and flakier, while the lower layer (the dermis) loses its substance and gets weak and lax, which promotes the wrinkling effect. Wrinkles occur also because the muscles underneath weaken. Over time our body's metabolism of the food we eat produces waste products that collect in our cells. The collection of toxins and metabolic junk, along with sun damage, will spur the appearance of benign growths such as seborrheic keratoses (little dirtlike, raised brown spots) and cherry angiomas (little red spots).

While these growths and other physical manifestations of age such as sagging skin are generally not harmful, they do reveal a reduced exchange of nutrients between the epidermis and the dermis. This is due to a reduced supply of blood to the area. How can you fight these issues?

Exercise. Followed by more exercise.

In a 2014 Canadian study detailed in the *New York Times*, twenty-nine volunteers aged twenty to eighty-four were asked to strip down and show a little derriere. This wasn't to be lewd, but to help researchers study a part of the skin that normally doesn't age due to exposure. After comparing the skin of twenty- and thirty-year-olds to that of the seniors, the researchers then asked people sixty-five and older who did not exercise to start moving those butts by using a simple, moderately strenuous, twice-a-week, thirty-minute cardio (jogging or cycling) program. When the study participants dropped their drawers three months later and had their skin rechecked, researchers found that the epidermal and dermal skin layers looked much like the skin of the twenty- to forty-year-olds.

When Is the Best Time to Exercise?

The quick answer is: whenever you find the time. Many people don't have time during the day due to work. It's a myth that exercising at night will keep you awake. In chapter 1, I mention that only about 3 percent of late exercisers have trouble sleeping as a result. Personally, I prefer to exercise in the morning, because there are advantages to doing so on an empty stomach. When you have fasted (meaning you haven't eaten for many hours), your insulin (the hormone that keeps blood sugar down) stays at a low level. Insulin helps drive the creation of fat in your body. When it is low, the ability to burn fat is higher—so you get more fat burning for your exercise buck!

Exercise Challenges and Solutions

Many patients I work with find certain challenges with exercise. I have listed the top ones here, and some solutions.

"I Can't Go Out in Bad Weather"

Many of my patients will say, "But it's cold and rainy. I can't go out today." Let me counter that objection quickly. I went to medical school with a woman who is now a colleague. When "Dr. Becky" invited me on my first camping trip, in the Oregon mountains, I protested: "I can't go. The weather is cold and rainy." Dr. Becky quickly replied, "Pina, there's no such thing as bad weather, just bad gear." Moral of the story: stop whining and buy some good outdoor exercise clothing—you know, that rainproof, windproof wicking material that keeps the warmth in and the rain out, while allowing your body to perspire. It will be money well spent. Equipped with that—barring ice, lightning, or other unsafe conditions—you're going out! And remember, spending time in nature will enhance your glow.

"No Time to Exercise; I'm at Work All Day"

You can do *something*, even at work. Remember, sitting is the new smoking. Just consider the recent rise in the use of the "standing desk." The only way to combat the deadly effects of not moving is by building time in your day to move. Set a timer to go off every twenty minutes to remind you to stand up and take a breath. In my office, I build in little breaks to take a walk around the block. If I can't get out, I do a quick burpee or two once an hour. A burpee is a four-step exercise movement in which you squat and place your hands on the floor, jump your feet back, bring them back to starting position, and then jump up in quick succession. It is a full-body move and really gets the blood going. Visit www.DrPinaND.com/burpee for a visual on how to do this.

"What If I Hate to Exercise?"

As a fellow human, I have to tell you, I have always struggled with exercise. I was a gymnast for years. I think that experience of always needing to be perfect and look perfect was a big part of my issue with irritable bowel syndrome and stress in my young age that contributed to the health problems I had for so many years. (For more on this, check out the box "Young Dr. Pina, Gymnast, and the Meaning of Life" in chapter 4.) When I stopped gymnastics, I shuddered at the thought of training for anything again.

Research has shown that unlike most men, most women don't enjoy exercise but do it to control weight and improve their appearance. This concerns me. When you use exercise as a means to an end rather than as a worthwhile process, you lose (or never experience) the joy of exercise for its own sake. In the long term, using exercise only to carve out what you perceive to be a younger- and skinnier-looking you can be more hurtful to your self-esteem. Your self-esteem is vitally important, and you need to protect and nourish it.

I want you to exercise to build your glow and stay healthy, not to add to a negative thought pattern. (If this resonates with you, you may want to jump to the next chapter, "Relaxation and Inner Peace," and see where those destructive thoughts are coming from.)

"What If I Physically Can't Exercise?"

Some people have physical ailments that don't allow them to exercise—for example, back pain, certain diseases, missing limbs, chronic fatigue, multiple sclerosis, or even heart failure. These are challenges that can be overcome—even patients with heart failure need to exercise.

At the University of Alberta in 2009, forty-two patients with heart failure were given an exercise regimen of both strength training and cardio three times a week for twelve weeks, at appropriate levels for each of them. Even these quite ill patients enjoyed clear increases in quality of life, strength, endurance, and cardiovascular health. If a heart failure patient can do it, you can do it, too. (Of course, it's important to check with your doctor before starting any exercise, to make sure it is right for your particular medical situation.)

Workouts That Work

....

We've briefly discussed the amazing benefits of exercise to health and looks, and we've troubleshot the main excuses. Now let's talk about what to do.

Some of you are already dedicated to exercise. Others might be new to the game. Welcome, both groups! What matters is that you're here and that you want to move. Let's talk about a few positive steps toward making exercise a regular part of your life. First we'll do cardio work, to get your body moving and your circulation going. Then we'll throw in some flexibility and balance work and finish with ways to sculpt your musculature. Exercise in this order will optimize results and reduce the chance of injury. (Of course, if you have any musculoskeletal limitations, talk to your doctor before starting any new kind of exercise.)

Exercise Step 1: Practice Cardio

Cardio, which is short for cardio- (aka heart) respiratory (aka lungs) fitness, is an easy way to start your glow juices flowing. Even if it's low impact, cardio is probably the best way to increase life expectancy and overall health. Cardio refers to any exercise that increases your heart and breathing rates. These two actions get more blood moving through your body, and more oxygen into more parts of your body.

Cardio to Prevent Cancer?

Cancer cells like an oxygen-deprived environment. Cardio exercise is the perfect way to increase circulation and bring oxygen to more areas. This is one of the reasons it will protect you from cancer.

If you haven't done cardio before, start with a walk three or four times a week. Make sure you wear a good pair of sneakers with excellent arch support. Don't be cheap—if your feet aren't well supported, your ankles, knees, hips, and a whole lot of other parts will suffer. If you are a runner, then thirty minutes four times a week is a healthy frequency for promoting longevity. If you have knee or back issues, try an elliptical machine or swimming for more comfort.

If you're new to running, start with three or four days a week of walking at a gentle pace for twenty minutes. Once this is comfortable, move up to forty minutes, and then even start a light jog here and there. If you like, you can work your way up to a forty-minute jog, but walking with only intermittent jogging is still great for elevating your heart rate. And, of course, simply walking is extremely beneficial to your body. Just make sure that it's a brisk walk, not a stroll.

Get your arms swinging and swaying. Singing "Dancing in the Street" is optional!

Exercise Step 2: Maintain Flexibility

Once you're warmed up from doing the cardio, it's a good time to do a little stretching. Particularly if you have blood sugar issues such as diabetes, warm-up and flexibility work are important ways to avoid exercise-induced injuries, because sugar glycation of tendons and ligaments will make them more prone to injury (see the section "Turn Down the Heat and Limit Your AGEs" in chapter 2 for more on this).

Simple hamstring, thigh, shoulder, lower back, and spine stretches for a few minutes will do the job. The best time to do these is after you've warmed up. Do them about eight to ten minutes after starting your cardio work, or at the end of the cardio. For more about these stretches, check out www.DrPinaND.com/flexibility.

Exercise Step 3: Achieve Balance

As women age, we have an increased danger of falling. I have seen many cases of patients whose history includes the unfortunate phrase "After I fell, my life was not the same." In most cases, falling can be prevented with the right balance exercises. *Proprioception* is a fancy word that refers to your brain's ability to know where a particular body part is in space, even when you're not looking at it. As we age, unless we are used to walking and working on uneven terrain, we tend to lose our proprioception and the use of the little auxiliary muscles that are needed to gently keep us upright and safe.

Balance work at any age will help you maintain or retain your proprioceptive competence. These exercises are simple. They take only a few minutes and can be done anywhere. Visit www.DrPinaND.com/balance to see videos, and download these and more easy exercises.

Balance Exercise *1*: Cross-Body Superwoman

While down on your knees, lift your right arm and left leg and hold for seven seconds; then lift your left arm and right leg and hold for seven seconds. Do this six times.

Balance Exercise *2*: DUI Test

First, find a straight line on the ground (twenty feet long is ideal) or create one of your own, maybe with blue painter's tape or chalk. Even better is a low "balance beam," such as the framed edge of a cobblestone path or a piece of lumber on the ground.

Walk with one foot right in front of the other, heel to toe, heel to toe. Take twenty-five steps like this. After step number twenty-five, swing your head and arms back in an "I stuck the landing!" pose, like Mary Lou Retton or Gabby Douglas used to do.

Balance Exercise 3: Tai Chi Primer

Tai chi has been studied by Harvard and many other institutions as a surefire way to strengthen balance and prevent falls, even in patients with Parkinson's disease. If it can help those with Parkinson's, it can help you, too. It is also shown to strengthen immunity, reduce pain, and aid sleep. Here are two exercises from the tai chi tradition:

Head Rolls

Stand with feet shoulder width apart, knees slightly bent. Relax and allow yourself to droop limply, like an overcooked piece of linguine. Inhale through the nose and raise your shoulders. Exhale through the mouth and lower your shoulders. Keep breathing and do two gentle head rolls: left, then right, and repeat.

Spread Your Wings

Standing straight with your arms by your sides, bring one knee up and to the side, holding it below your ribs so that the foot is hovering alongside your supporting knee but not resting on it. Then, with palms facing down, raise your arms straight out to the side, above your shoulders, as if you're a bird. Hold for three seconds while breathing. Then lower your arms, switch legs, and bring your arms back up. Do this ten times.

If you are concerned about falling, you may want

to have someone with you for the first few times you try these exercises.

Balance Exercise *4*: Build Muscle

So we moved through cardio, flexibility, and balance. That is a good setup for starting to build muscle. Keeping good muscle composition is a primary way to prevent diabetes, heart disease, cancer, and osteoporosis. In 2012 the Oregon Health and Science University studied strength training effects on 106 postmenopausal breast cancer patients who had already undergone radiation and chemotherapy treatments. Building muscle showed astonishing benefits in preventing bone loss and decreasing the side effects of aromatase inhibitor drugs (e.g., tamoxifen), which rob the body of muscle-maintaining hormones. Other studies have shown that breast cancer survivors who exercise greatly reduce the likelihood of breast cancer recurrence.

I've seen this story replicated with many, many patients. While supplements are helpful in building bone, they don't work without the exercise. You need the exercise and resistance training to "remodel" and strengthen your bones. We tend to view bones as kind of hard and dead, but in actuality they're living tissue, and they need the circulation and challenge that exercise provides.

If you're new to exercise, I strongly recommend working with a knowledgeable trainer. Ask your fit friends whom they work with. You may think it's too expensive. Believe me, any money you spend on your trainer is money you'll save on trips to the doctor down the line. It is worth it.

Case: Lauren with Diabetes

Lauren, a patient with brittle diabetes (an advanced form of the condition that is considered hard to treat), came into my clinic because her blood sugar levels were around 300 milligrams per deciliter (normal is about 80 to 95), and her hemoglobin A1c (a measure of blood sugar over three months) was very high at 8.2 (5.8 and above is usually associated with diabetes). Lauren's blood produced these numbers despite the fact that she was on two medications to lower them. She came in wanting "herbs to lower blood sugar." I let her know that I would work with herbs, but I needed also to bring in diet changes and exercise. Lauren said that she'd be willing to work on the food, but exercise was "out" because she was too dizzy even to walk; her doctors had said that exercise was too dangerous. I believed her, for I saw her walk slowly, dragging her feet and holding on to her husband—she was ready to fall at any moment.

Obviously, going for a jog was out. So we started with a tabletop pedal machine (twenty bucks at Amazon—I love a good deal!). Her endocrinologist agreed (reluctantly) to this. Lauren used the machine for five minutes three times a day—nice and easy. As we worked on the food and started her on the herbs, we increased the exercise slowly. Within two months, Lauren had graduated to a recumbent bike. After four months, her A1c was down to 7.5, and her blood sugars hovered around 180. Within eight months, she was walking outdoors, with a blood sugar of 120 and an A1c of 5.8, and using only one medication at a low dose.

Chapter 4

RELAXATION AND INNER PEACE

Healing is possible even in the absence of cure.

Cure is about the recovery of the body.

Healing is about the recovery of the soul.

—RACHEL NAOMI REMEN, HOLISTIC PHYSICIAN AND AUTHOR

uter beauty and health are indicators of what goes on inside your body. So far, this book has addressed sleep, food, and exercise to help guide you to your most radiant self. Perhaps you're stressed and may even be depressed—25 percent of Americans experience one or both. In my New York practice, it is the rare patient who is not on an antianxiety or antidepressant medication.

There's a better way to beat stress and the blues: inner peace.

Telling someone to cultivate inner peace is kind of like telling someone, "Just be perfect." Okay, let me put that on my shopping list: a pound of salmon, toilet paper, oh, and pick up some inner peace.

So, let's start by getting one basic concept ironed out right now: Inner peace isn't something you'll ever attain completely. It is something you move toward; it's an ideal, and the journey is what's important.

To help you move toward that ideal, in this chapter we are going to talk about two things: relaxation methods to cultivate peace so your body and mind calm, and how to change the thoughts that can derail true serenity.

Suffering from a Low Mood or Depression?

Follow these steps to start feeling better quickly. (You can safely do these while continuing your medication.)

1. **Take a multivitamin.** Vitamins are molecules that help your body make the neurotransmitters it needs. Follow the dosage on the bottle and take with food.

2. **Take fish oil.** Fish oil helps keep the brain and nerves in better shape. Look for a dose of

1,000 mg of eicosapentaenoic acid (EPA) per day

3. **Take vitamin D₃.** Known as the "happy vitamin," vitamin D_3 should be taken in one 1,000 IU dose a day with food. Ask your doctor to test your levels.

4. **Get more sunlight and exercise.** Spending time outdoors, moving the body, is a powerful antidepressant.

5. **Get a full eight hours of sleep.** Sleep is crucial for both your outer *and* inner well-being.

If you are thinking even remotely of hurting yourself, **reach out and get help**. At the National Suicide Prevention Center Lifeline, at 1-800-273-TALK (8255), there are many people waiting to help you.

Relaxation

There are many wonderful ways to create and cultivate an environment for your self-esteem and bliss. We are going to talk about my favorites: spending time in nature, meditating, getting acupuncture, and receiving massage work. Solid research backs claims of how healthy and effective these are. Their benefits will show in your glowing face.

Relaxation Method 1: Spend Time in Nature

One of the main tenets of naturopathic medicine is that nature heals your body and helps it return to the balance it was meant for. To do this, simply bathe your body in a natural environment where there are trees, plants, sky above, and fresh air. You and I are really just animals, and animals need to be in nature to stay healthy.

The Japanese reverence for nature takes form in a practice called *shinrin-yoku*, or "forest bathing." Studies of seniors show that forest bathing lowers heart rate and blood pressure and reduces inflammation. I'm sure you've heard the word *inflammation* tossed around quite a bit. Keep in mind that it should never be discounted; inflammation is a nasty contributor to pretty much *all* disease.

✳ Studies of hospitalized patients show that those who have a view of nature from their recovery rooms experience less post-surgery pain and anxiety, ditch their painkillers sooner, and recover faster. Also, people who viewed abstract art after surgery actually had *more* anxiety than those who stared at a blank wall. Maybe the abstract art had too many unnatural-looking lines that caused stress for them at a primitive brain level. For our health, Mother Nature is the best interior designer.

Try to schedule at least three days a week during which you can spend twenty minutes in a park or forest. If you can't make the time, at least sit near an open window that looks out on trees and plants. Your soul will feel it.

Nature can be brought indoors, too. In one study, participants who held a houseplant for two minutes were calmer and showed less brain stress. Other studies show that just having plants in a room can lower blood pressure. Patients tell me their blood pressure drops in my office versus when they are in other doctors' offices. I thought it was my charm, but maybe it's my plants. While all plants can help calm the environment, in the next chapter ("Detoxification"), I will mention plants especially good for cleaning the air in your home, too, so look for these.

Relaxation Method 2: Meditate

> *Meditation is about being yourself and knowing who that is.*
>
> —JON KABAT-ZINN, FOUNDER OF
> MINDFULNESS-BASED STRESS REDUCTION

Dating back to 2000 BCE, meditation was first mentioned in the Vedas, the early writings that documented Ayurvedic medicine, the most ancient known medical system in the world. There are various forms of meditation, such as yogic, Zen, mindfulness, and Transcendental Meditation.

Just as everyone should drink plenty of water, everyone should meditate. The transformation I witness when patients start to meditate is fascinating. People sleep better, think more clearly, and are better able to handle the challenges of life.

✳ Meditation has been shown, in well-designed trials, to improve psychological stress responses; lower anxiety, depression, and anger; balance blood pressure while lowering risk of heart attack and stroke; and greatly reduce chronic pain. Studies suggest that it may even help slow the aging process. Meditation has demonstrated an ability to improve telomere length, which is a secret to living longer. Telomeres are protective caps to our DNA, and the shorter they become, the faster we age (more about these gene protectors in the next chapter).

How to Meditate

1. Pick a time of day to sit in a relaxed way—morning is great, for it sets a calm tone for the day.

2. Breathe from your belly. Generally, you should breathe in through your nose and out through your mouth.

3. When you breathe in, visualize your belly filling with beautiful, calming air that is

sending oxygen through your whole body. Then gently breathe out and visualize that you are expelling into the universe all that you don't need, to be recycled into positive energy.

You can meditate for thirty seconds, five minutes, or as long as you like, really. If you haven't meditated before, start with brief sessions, continuing for longer as it feels right.

Tip: Set your smartphone timer to go off with a nice, calming alarm, to bring you back to the present moment. There are many phone apps available for meditation.

Often when you meditate, you will find your thoughts trying to butt in. That's okay. Just move back to your breath. If a particular thought is especially bothersome, write it down and then return to your breathing. You can look at it later to see what issues require your attention.

If you need help, please visit www.DrPinaND .com/meditation to find a basic guided meditation audio track to follow.

Relaxation Method *3: Consult an Acupuncturist*

I love acupuncture—so much so that I decided to earn a master's degree in it while doing my medical training. Even though I've practiced acupuncture for eleven years, I'm still amazed by how well it works.

✳ The World Health Organization has documented the effectiveness of acupuncture in treating more than 250 diseases. The evidence points to its ability to slow the body's molecular events associated with getting older: stimulating certain points can reverse the natural genetic tendency of the brain's hippocampus to age. (The hippocampus is the emotional and memory center in the brain.) The points studied included Stomach 36 (a point on the leg known to help the digestive tract and immune system) and Conception Vessel 17 (a point right smack in between your breasts, on the breastbone). Conception Vessel 17 is good for the heart, breast issues, and overall energy. A 2007 review of twelve studies found that acupuncture delivered very positive results in the treatment of both generalized anxiety disorder and neurosis (a milder form of chronic anxiety). Auricular (outside ear) acupuncture was especially useful for keeping people calm before surgical procedures.

How Does Acupuncture Work?

Acupuncture involves inserting fine needles into various spots on the body, first to balance your yin and yang energy and then to balance you with the environment around you. Yin is the dark, cool, Mother Earth, female energy. Yang is the light, warm, energetic, male energy we all have inside us. In Chinese medicine, when these are out of balance, deficient, or excessive, disease can follow.

Does Acupuncture Hurt, and Is It Safe?

I have many patients who were at first afraid of acupuncture, only to find that it's calming and relaxing. The needles do *not* hurt. They feel like a pin stick that goes away quickly. Occasionally, you may feel a dull ache—nothing dramatic—but if for some reason you feel pain, tell your acupuncturist, and she'll remove the needle pronto. Acupuncture is very safe when performed by a professional; it does not adversely interact with other treatments, such as drugs. It's also safe during pregnancy and for women who are breast-feeding. Large-scale studies have reviewed millions of acupuncture treatments and found exceedingly rare side effects.

So, get thee to an acupuncturist! Usually I recommend starting with sessions twice a week, and once you're feeling better, move to once a week for maintenance.

Relaxation Method 4: Get a Massage

Like Chinese medicine, massage has very ancient beginnings. Hippocrates, the father of medicine, taught all his medical students the benefits of "rubbing" to increase circulation and heal the body. In naturopathic school, we students were given a massage class, where we learned proper technique. This was really tough (wink wink), because we also had to act as guinea pigs for our fellow classmates. That was my favorite class!

✳ In the 1990s, a series of studies showed how massage increases a sense of peace and lowers levels of the stress hormone cortisol while simultaneously increasing the feel-good neurotransmitters dopamine and serotonin. In addition, almost 80 percent of patients experienced a significant reduction in anxiety. These results are similar to those achieved through psychotherapy. I imagine that with both treatments combined, the numbers would only improve.

Here's a tough prescription: take one for the team and go get a nice relaxation massage. It's easy to find well-trained, accredited, licensed massage therapists through the American Massage Therapy Association, at www.amtamassage.org.

Types of Massage

- Swedish: uses light to medium pressure;
- Deep tissue: good for muscle tension and knots;
- Reflexology: focuses on hands and feet, to calm the body;
- Cranialsacral: very light and gentle; great for osteoporotic women; and
- Shiatsu: light; based on Asian medicine principles.

Inner Peace

Okay—you've spent time in nature, meditated, had some acupuncture, and gotten a massage. Let's hope you're feeling a little more Zen than before. Now I would like to touch on the thoughts that can cultivate inner peace, or chase it away.

Many of my patients are bravely slogging on through life but are not truly happy. If this describes you, please take your time with the next section—and remember, a calm brain will translate into a body with a more balanced physiology, less inflammation, less disease, a slower aging process, and, most important, a happy brain.

Three Important Questions for Inner Peace

When I work with a patient of any age or either gender, I ask these questions:

1. Do you have a good sense of self-esteem?

2. Are there aspects of your life that you feel passionate about?

3. Do you purposefully and regularly help others?

I think about the questions in that order, as one answer enriches the next. To think about it graphically (this one can go on your fridge):

> ✎ build your self-esteem
> ✎ follow your passions
> ✎ help others with their journey

Let me explain further: A good sense of self-esteem gives you the courage to follow what is important to you. Poor self-esteem is often at the root of fear. When you believe in yourself, you can go out and follow the road you believe you were destined for, whether that's playing in a band, being a lawyer, driving a truck, staying home with the kids, staying single . . . anything. When self-esteem is poor, we sometimes make choices based on what feels safest, as opposed to what our heart spirit is saying. This will often lead to greater stress, anxiety, and even depression.

I also believe that when your spirit is not allowed to manifest, it can lead to whatever physical illness you may be predisposed to. Once we are following our passions, often we like to help others to do the same. For example, I love having aspiring students in my clinic—I love what I do, and I love to share it. This book is a manifestation of that spirit. My great hope is that there will be something in here that will connect with you and help your life.

Steps Toward Greater Self-Esteem

So, how do you start working on self-esteem? As just mentioned, poor self-esteem is correlated with fear. The way to deal with fear? Check in with the messages you tell yourself.

Self-Esteem Step *1*: Recognize and Change Negative Thoughts

To risk sounding like an old Whitney Houston tune, the greatest love of all really is loving yourself. Maybe you've heard this; maybe you're even tired of hearing it. But you have to face it. It is the truth.

With the scores of women I have worked with, and in my own life, I have found self-esteem to be the greatest challenge. I see girls in their teens who feel they don't fit in, women in their twenties and thirties who want to prove themselves, women in their forties who never found the right partner and still desperately want a child, women in their fifties and beyond who lived the life they were told to and are now questioning whether they are actually happy. Does any of this sound familiar?

Many women love being parents, they like their work, and they do a lot for others, but their self-esteem is still low. The problem is if you're not happy with yourself, there's no way you can be truly happy with another person, or with anything else in life. At any age.

Earlier we talked about exercise. Later we are going to talk about vitamins. I see how some women use exercise only to carve out the "perfect" appearance, or vitamins to keep themselves looking younger. That can be more hurtful than helpful to your self-esteem because it establishes the idea that only when you reach a certain dress size, weight, or cup size, or when you achieve a wrinkle-free appearance or the absence of gray hair, will you be happy. This strips your self-esteem by giving you specific parameters that define who you are and your happiness.

Here's a tip: what you think about yourself is more important and more valuable than any particular measurement, look, or parameter someone else can assign you.

Most of what I talk about in this book revolves around physical health. I talk about the right foods to eat, how to cook, exercise, take vitamins, and so on. What's the point of all this? Is it to be perfect with your food intake and know the best vitamins? Not at all. The point of all this to-do to make yourself healthier is so that you can go out and live who you really are and what your spirit proclaims—and then help others. That to me is true health.

Young Dr. Pina, Gymnast, and the Meaning of Life

When I was younger I was a gymnast. I was pretty good at it, too. In fact, when I was nine years old, my trainer wanted to send me to train at the camp run by famous coach Béla Károlyi, just outside Houston. That's a place where many of the future Olympians train. As you might expect, immigrant Sicilian moms living in New York don't really like seeing their daughters head off to Texas indefinitely, so that Olympic dream was nixed.

One thing I learned from my gymnastics work is that if you are looking for perfection all the time, you will not get it. In gymnastics, I was taught to be a ten, or to go home. For a long time I was consistently unhappy with my gymnastics; I always felt I could be better. No matter how good I became (and I was very good), no matter how many awards and competitions I won, I remained unhappy. Why? Because instead of enjoying the moment, I was always looking for the next big thing or focusing on what had gone wrong or could go wrong. Now I know that's not the way to live, or grow.

I love my mom tremendously. However, as no parent is perfect, she unintentionally passed down some negative ideas about how I should think about myself (which were lovingly ingrained in her by *her* mom, my *nonna*). Ah, Italian guilt—the gift that keeps on giving. My mom taught me early on not to show my body at all. And she taught that if I didn't have at least some makeup on my face, I wouldn't look good. And I believed her.

Yet I took it to a new level—in my mind, I was never good enough in any way: not how I looked, not in my gymnastics, not in my academic work. It's funny, I've appeared on TV shows as a health and wellness expert more times than I can count, but at some level, I still feel like I don't know enough, don't look good, and have little to offer, even though the world tells me otherwise.

You see, I am still working on my self-esteem—

and I want you to work on yours. It's the most important work we can do.

So, what do we do now?

If you have ever been involved with addiction work, you know that the first step to recovering from alcoholism is acknowledging that you're drinking too much and noticing when you're doing it. When people are genuinely addicted to alcohol, they typically don't realize how often or how much they drink. Similarly, you may be addicted to negative thoughts and low self-esteem.

In her wonderful work *When Things Fall Apart*, Pema Chödrön writes, "Rather than letting our negativity get the better of us, we could acknowledge that right now we feel like a piece of shit and not be squeamish about taking a good look."

How do you rise above the idea of not ever being good enough?

1. Acknowledge that you are addicted to negative thinking.

2. Look at yourself gently and with compassion and challenge those thoughts. Ask yourself: How would you treat your best friend if you noticed she was beating herself up all the time? What would you tell her? You would probably very gently tell her to stop those thoughts because they are misguided. You

might ask her to be kinder to herself. *This* is how you need to talk to yourself.

3. Write 'em down. As an exercise, when you catch yourself having negative thoughts about yourself, I'd like you to start writing them down. Then recast each thought in a positive way. Finally, think the new, positive thought, even if you don't mean it. In time, you will get used to your new truths:

    Current thought: I look old.
    New thought: I look the way I need to right now, and I am working on my best health.
    Current thought: I am unhealthy.
    New thought: My body is giving me signs to help me make better choices.
    Current thought: I hate my boss.
    New thought: As I open my heart, I know that my boss is placed here as a teacher for me.
    Current thought: I am a bad mother.
    New thought: Overall, I am a good mom and I am doing my best every day.

As you practice this, you will find it gets easier. I also strongly recommend that during this process, you read works with positive messages, such as Pema Chödrön's wonderful books (they are all good), to help you reframe the negativity and move yourself forward positively.

If you want to go further with this, Dr. Carolyn Myss, Marianne Williamson, and Mastin Kipp have all written wonderful works on self-esteem and changing negative thought patterns.

Self-Esteem Step 2: Follow Your Passions

Joseph Campbell was a brilliant mythologist and teacher at Sarah Lawrence College. My husband, Peter, introduced me to Campbell's work, and I was immediately fascinated. Campbell spent his life researching ancient civilizations, such as those of the Mayans and Egyptians, to study their belief systems. He also learned a great deal from writers of literature such as James Joyce and Shakespeare. Something he found common to all these cultures was the idea of the "hero's journey." Campbell's famous advice regarding a successful hero's journey was to "follow your bliss."

We are all on a hero's journey. You are—as were the great figures in religion (think Buddha, Jesus, and Muhammad), in pop art (think Superman), and in popular cartoons (think Disney's Mulan, one of my favorite female characters of all time).

If your self-esteem is strong, you will move toward doing the things that make you happy. This isn't selfish; it is following your bliss.

So, in this second step, ask yourself this: "What are my passions? What makes my heart sing?"

What If I Don't Know What My Passions Are?

Now, you might be thinking, "I don't know what my passions are; that is the problem." This is totally okay. It just means now is the opportunity to start listening further. Really listen. This is one of the purposes of meditation and even a step toward getting healthy and detoxing.

Take a moment to write your passions down. Yes, physically write them down—don't just think about them. There is a big difference in how the brain processes something you merely think about as opposed to something you commit to paper, so the act of writing is important here. Maybe your passion is playing a musical instrument, learning to cook, painting in watercolors, or working as a veterinarian. These could be hobbies, careers, or avocations. The important thing is to list them, and to look at them objectively.

No matter how wacky or unrealistic your passion, write it down. Then share it with people you trust. Sharing it with good people will start the brainstorming process. Brainstorming with others, talking about your passion, is the first step to making it real. Ask the people you share with to help you create an action list.

Start simple. For example, take a class in your area of interest. See where it leads you.

What If There Are Obstacles to Following My Passions?

Maybe you can't leave your kids or job to go to cooking school and become a gourmet chef, but maybe you *can* take a weekend cooking class for a Saturday or two. The heart doesn't care about titles or whether you become a professional. And you may not be in a position to create an income from your passion. That's okay. Your heart just wants you to go after something you're passionate about.

If you are still stuck and don't know what your passion might be, that's okay, too. No pressure. Just move through the rest of this book. Getting healthier in other ways can help open up the brain and lead you to the answers you're seeking. Also, you may want to consider individualized help by working with a naturopathic doctor, or find a good life coach who can support you through the process.

Remember, it's never too late to find a passion! I have patients who started skiing, painting, running marathons, and studying instruments in their seventies and eighties. You should see their smiles and experience their sense of pride. That's living life passionately.

Self-Esteem Step 3: Help Others with Their Journeys

If you want others to be happy, practice compassion.
If you want to be happy, practice compassion.

—DALAI LAMA

We are all connected to one universal energy. You are not in this alone. Since our energies are connected, what helps or hurts one of us affects the rest of us. In this spirit, part of our journey here is to assist others with their journeys.

There are many ways to do this. It might be by doing charity work, such as volunteering at a soup kitchen or giving a portion of what you earn for someone else's well-being. One of my patients anonymously donated money to send a boy to a school he couldn't otherwise afford. Your contribution can be more active than that, such as working in a job that directly helps people with their lives (for example, as a nurse or teacher). There are many noble pursuits.

The first step to helping others with their journeys could be even simpler. It could involve your mindfulness, making an effort to thank the people in your life who support you and being more conscious of how you treat others. Or maybe simply smile more and give people compliments. People love to receive compliments, and it feels good to give them.

Higher Power—Yea or Nay?

Whether we call him or her God, Allah, Yahweh, Mother Earth, Vishnu, Krishna, Divine Mother, or Universal Energy, it's been shown that people who connect to a higher power have less depression and anxiety, fare better with medical treatments for disease, and are less vulnerable to emotional distress in times of physical illness. Belief systems often come with a host of conflicting ideologies and can cause alienation. But when a belief system resonates with you, it can also bring you closer to others—and to the person you really are, in terms of the spirit you have been nourishing. If belief in a higher power is something that resonates with you, then I say go for it.

Chapter 5

DETOXIFICATION

I cannot put this poison on my skin.
I do not use anything synthetic.

—GISELE BÜNDCHEN, SUPERMODEL

Every year, almost 90,000 new chemicals are registered with the U.S. government. Also each year, about 4 billion pounds of toxic chemicals are released into the nation's environment. In 2009 the U.S. Centers for Disease Control delivered its most comprehensive report on environmental exposure to common chemicals. Studying 2,400 individuals, CDC researchers learned that most Americans have more than 212 toxins weighing them down. And there's nowhere to run; you can leave the United States, but these chemicals have been found pretty much everywhere in the world. Even 22,000 feet up, on the peaks of the Andes.

Researchers at two major laboratories found an average of 200 industrial chemicals and pollutants in cord blood, the blood in the umbilical cord connecting a pregnant mother to her baby. Of the 287 chemicals detected in cord blood, 180 of them can cause cancer in humans or animals, 217 are toxic to the brain and nervous system, and 208 have been shown to cause birth defects or abnormal development in animal tests.

Reams of solid research now show that people age much faster when there are foreign chemicals present in the body's tissue.

Yikes!

Don't worry, though. While much of it sounds like doom and gloom, I am not providing this information to scare you. Instead, it is to empower you, for knowledge is power. And knowledge and education are the keys to understanding how to fix this challenge.

The first part of this chapter will help you identify (sometimes in too much detail) the toxins and their sources. The second half will take you through my method of detoxification, giving you practical ways to prevent exposure and help you usher those toxins out of your body.

Why Are Some People Sensitive to Chemicals While Others Are Not?

Scientists still don't know why some people react to toxins more than others. It is likely that some people's bodies are equipped either to detoxify chemicals or safely store nasty molecules in certain bodily tissues (e.g., in the fat and bone), thus keeping the toxins away from more active tissues and organs. So the same level of toxic exposure that can wreak havoc on one person may have little or no effect on another.

The Signs and Symptoms of Toxicity

While toxic burden can mimic virtually any disease, the most common signs and symptoms of toxicity are:

- dullness in the eyes;
- blemishes and age spots;
- bloating;
- hormonal ups and downs;
- nervous system problems;
- heart disease;

- cancer;
- excessive wrinkles;
- fatigue for no apparent reason;
- excessive fat tissue under the skin;
- fatty liver disease (also called nonalcoholic liver steatosis);
- diabetes or high blood sugar;
- high GGT (a liver test) and high liver enzymes; and
- high levels of mercury and other toxins in the blood.

If you have any of these signs and symptoms, it is important to have your doctor do a proper workup. In most cases, conventional medicine will find no clear reason for them. This is the time to think about detoxification—for it is likely that the body wants to clean house, inside and out.

❋ Telomeres

A 2014 paper by researchers at the University of North Carolina clearly shows that many everyday environmental toxins accelerate the aging process. This work explains how researchers are using new technology that scans telomeres, the ends of your genetic material. Telomeres remind me of the plastic thingy at the tip of your shoelace, the aglet. What happens if that aglet breaks? The shoelace frays, which makes it pretty unusable and susceptible to more damage. Similarly, toxins in our environment will break the protective tips of our genes and cause the genetic material to fray and become exposed. This leads to the malfunctioning and aging of our cells while predisposing us to a host of diseases, including cancer and heart disease. The Mediterranean diet (see chapter 2) keeps your genetic material intact by keeping your telomeres healthy and strong. A study of more than 121,000 people tracked since 1996 looked at how following a Mediterranean diet can maintain telomere health. Likely, a good diet like the Mediterranean plan will lower your toxic intake and help you usher toxins safely out of your body.

What Causes Telomeres to Shorten?

- poor nutrition
- lack of sleep
- overeating
- low vitamin D
- stress

Gerontogens: Chemicals That Age Us Faster

According to German researcher Paraskevi Gkogko-lou, of the University of Münster, aging is defined as the "progressive accumulation of damage to an organism over time leading to disease and death." What causes this damage? Chemical toxins from our environment and our own metabolic processes cause aging reactions in our bodies.

That all of us are inundated with nasty age-accelerating chemicals isn't news. In 1987, University of Washington aging expert Dr. George Martin coined the term *gerontogen* (from the Greek *geron*, meaning "old man"). He was the first person to assign a name to the chemicals in our environment that prematurely age the body. Dr. Martin also recognized that the natural pace of aging, which is determined by our genes, can be highly accelerated by exposure to chemicals foreign to our bodies.

Please, Don't Yell at the Kids

Research has shown that children who are regularly yelled at have shorter telomeres relative to their peers who live in gentler household environments.

The Keith Richards Effect

For years we have noticed that people who have smoked a lot of cigarettes and/or taken a lot of recreational drugs look much older than their actual age. (My musician husband calls this the Keith Richards effect.) They are also more likely to develop cancer, cardiovascular disease, and other chronic diseases. Dr. Martin realized that the hundreds of chemicals in cigarettes and other recreational drugs are not the only ones that make us look older. The chemicals that various industries expel into the seas and air and the ones put in our food have very similar aging effects. These effects might be slower and less obvious than those caused by cigarettes and street drugs, but they are real, and are definitely aging our bodies from the inside out.

Common Gerontogens

While there are more gerontogens than I could possibly mention in this chapter, I am going to talk about a few major ones. It is important for you to know how these show up and function in your environment and body so that you can avoid them.

As you read this next section, please remember that the second part of the chapter will explain how to limit your accumulation of damage.

Cigarettes

Vanity can save a life! The number one reason women stop smoking is because smoking causes wrinkles. This is a no-brainer—if you are reading this book, you likely already know that cigarettes age you, are the number one cause of cancer, cause heart disease, and will amp up pretty much every disease to which you may be predisposed. Regular smokers die, on average, seven years younger than nonsmokers. Smoking also destroys gene-protecting telomeres. Besides avoiding smoking, look out for secondhand smoke (breathing in other people's smoke) and thirdhand smoke, the smoke released from other people's clothing, carpeting, and so on. The "Detoxification Process" section will offer advice on how to quit smoking.

Chemical Toxins

Besides the ubiquity of cigarette smoke, another environmental concern is crazy chemical assaults that lead to aging, poor health, and the general dimming of your beautiful glow. These affronts often come from the use of plastics, insecticides, herbicides, paints, wood preservatives, sanitizers, and the thousands of other industrial and household chemicals to which we're exposed. These chemicals cause the liver to function poorly, which can lead to obesity and hormonal dysregulation, diabetes, and cancer.

✳ Known as endocrine (hormonal) disruptors, **organotins** are widely used in industry to stop fungal and bacterial growth and to keep away rodents. In one study of a polluted lake, female fish were shown to become more masculine due to exposure to organotins. In women, organotins cause liver toxicity, obesity, and hormonal dysregulation. **Parabens** are used as preservatives in many cosmetic products, including lotions, creams, and shampoos. They also bind to hormone receptors in the body. Studies from 2004 and 2011 show that breast cancer occurs more often in the outer quadrant of the breast. This is the area of the underarm where cosmetic products such as antiperspirants and deodorants are typically applied. Even more, breast tumor biopsies have all found parabens in the cancer tissue. While these studies do not prove that parabens cause cancer, my thought is to avoid them just in case.

Plastics line our food packaging, water pipes, and medical tubing, and even flake off our cash register receipts. It's been documented that male workers in factories that produce receipts and men who regularly handle receipts have lower levels of testosterone and poor sperm count. Low testosterone levels are associated with the inability to maintain muscle tone and sexual interest, and lead to premature aging. **Bisphenols** are a type of hormone disruptor present in most plastics. One type of bisphenol is bisphenol A (BPA). Another common plasticizer is **phthalates**, which are melded into food packaging. The most common house-hold sources of phthalates, however, are lotions, per-fumes, and cosmetics. Unless you are choosing super-clean organic cosmetics, the products you're using to keep yourself looking young might be aging you. Now banned due to neurological toxicity, **polychlorinated biphenyls (PCBs)** are chlorine- and benzene-based molecules ubiquitous in electrical industry parts, car-bonless paper, and industrial fluids.

Persistent organic pollutants (POPs) include many insecticides, pesticides, herbicides, and dioxin. In 2006 the journal *Diabetes Care* published a land-mark study showing that people who had higher lev-els of POPs in their urine were much more likely to develop diabetes, whether or not they were obese. This is shocking, for it has long been believed that obesity is the main risk factor for diabetes. Now we are learning that the presence of toxins is also a cul-prit. People with diabetes clearly age quicker, become frail, and look much older than their years. Use of these poisons also correlates with mental frailty and much higher levels of anxiety and suicide. So these chemicals age us *and* make us unhappy in the process.

Heavy metals such as arsenic, cadmium, mer-cury, aluminum, and lead are found in dental amal-gams, welding, cigarettes, galvanized water pipes, and even some foods. Heavy metals lead to clear destruc-tive, aging changes in your body. These raise blood pressure and stress the cardiovascular system. Arsenic has potent cancer-causing epigenetic effects. Heavy metals deplete antioxidant reserves, which leads to inflammatory reactions and oxidative stress. Oxidative stress ages your skin by using up the nutrients that fight to keep it hydrated and looking young. Heavy metals also inhibit the normal metabolic workings of the cell by destroying the mitochondria, the energy-making centers for every cell in your body.

Natural Supplements May Not Be Safe, Either

Even natural medicines have been contaminated with metal toxicities. Two separate studies found that herbs from both India (called Ayurvedic herbs) and China were contaminated and caused exposure to heavy metals in the people who took them. This is a reason to use supplements and herbs you know are processed with the most stringent testing, of both the raw materials and the finished supplement product. If you do not know which ones these are, work with a naturopathic doctor or other knowledgeable practitioner who understands supplement quality and can help you wade through the marketing and labeling hype.

If These Chemicals Are So Dangerous, Why Isn't the Government Protecting Us?

Environmental research reveals that toxic exposures accumulate slowly, and insidiously, over long periods of time, and cause slow degeneration of the body. So they can't be pinned down by studies to prove their deadly effects absolutely. Europeans won't use chemicals unless they are proven safe, but in the United States, we allow their use until they are proven *unsafe*. As a result, we have nefarious molecules in our air, food, and water.

Medications

While medications can be lifesaving when used in appropriate urgent-care situations, they can also be toxic. According *The Journal of the American Medical Association*, properly prescribed medications have strong effects on the body that suppress symptoms, which helps us feel better, but can cause many medical problems, and even lead to death. Medications also contain binders, fillers, and colors (such as tartrazine and other dyes) with toxic profiles that create free radical production and inflammatory responses of their own. As you read the section "The Detoxification

Process," later in this chapter, remember that it's important not to make any changes to your medication dosage without consulting your prescribing physician first.

Mold

Mold spores are floating through the air all the time, and sometimes these little guys will find a nice damp, dark, out-of-the-way place where they collect toxins and grow into full-blown toxic mold. Toxic mold elements, called mycotoxins, can wreak havoc on your immune system, creating chronic inflammation that ages you and makes you more susceptible to many other illnesses, including chronic fatigue, heart disease, asthma, and dementia.

An estimated 4.6 million cases of asthma are caused by mold. Also, it is likely many more people are completely unaware that mold is the cause of their health problems. Conventionally trained medical doctors learn very little about mycology (the study of mold) in medical school. Dr. Ritchie Shoemaker was one of the first doctors to study mold, and his work reveals that about 25 percent of people are especially susceptible to illness from toxic mold. Later in this chapter, we will talk about how to test for these noxious fungi, and which tests you need to determine if mold is contributing to aging and illness in your life.

Air Pollution

Breathing is the easiest and fastest way to get unwanted dangerous chemicals into your body. The job of the lungs is to get precious oxygen into our cells to help make energy. Since this is so vital, the lungs created a system that allows air to have easy access to the bloodstream. The lung cells use the air we breathe to help deliver oxygen right to the red blood cells. There is nothing in between to act as a filter. This is by design: if oxygen can't get to the red blood cells, we suffocate. Unfortunately, any toxin in the air will get in there, too, right into our bloodstream. It is as if we've placed an IV in our arm to let the toxic compounds drip right in. You know when you buy a vinyl curtain for your shower, and that new vinyl smell emanates from it? That vinyl is going right into your bloodstream. It's the same with chlorine vapors from warmed shower mist.

According to the American Heart Association, air pollution poses a serious threat to cardiovascular (and overall) health, with burning fossil fuels and diesel particulates creating inflammatory reactions that cause chronic inflammation and overall increased mortality.

Inflammation ages us. Overactive immune cells end up destroying other healthy tissue in the body, leading to chronic disease and aging. The blood vessels also get mucked up, causing poor circulation to the skin and low flow to vital organs, and stealing needed oxygen from the heart. In the "Detoxification Process" section, we will talk about how to ward off this pollution and thus lower inflammation in our bodies.

Drinking Water

Ah, H_2O—the most natural substance for your body. We are composed mostly of water. So it makes sense that the water we're drinking will impact how healthy we are. Numerous pharmaceuticals, pesticides, herbicides, heavy metals, POPs, and plastics are found in our water supply.

It's not bad enough that our water is polluted, but we then treat it with even more chemicals, in an effort to "clean" it. In this process, we add perchlorates (chlorine compounds) that inhibit thyroid function and oxidize the fats in our bloodstream. Poor thyroid function and lipid oxidation are contributors to aging. We also add chlorine, which turns to chloroform. You may recognize chloroform from old movies—the bad guy would soak a handkerchief with it and hold the cloth over the good guy's mouth to knock him unconscious. Well, small amounts of it in our drinking water damage our nervous system while aging us at the same time.

Most Polluted Drinking Water, by State*

- Arizona
- California
- Florida
- Illinois
- Nevada
- New York
- North Carolina
- Pennsylvania
- Texas
- Wisconsin

* In alphabetical order

Is Fluoride Safe?

Many experts consider fluoride to be "forced medication." It's unproven in preventing cavities, and studies from India link fluoride exposure to bone cancer. It has also been linked to increases in bone and hip fractures, birth defects, prenatal deaths, and lead and arsenic exposure. On top of that, it suppresses your thyroid function. As a result, many countries have banned water fluoridation. According to data published in the July 2009 *Journal of the American Dental Association*, children living in areas where the water is not fluoridated develop about the same number of cavities as children living in areas with fluoridation. In 2006 the National Academy of Sciences published a report titled *Fluoride in Drinking Water: A Scientific Review of EPA Standard,* which indicated that fluoride is simply not necessary. So, why the heck are we poisoning ourselves with this stuff?

What About Bottled Water?

Unless your water is bottled in glass, it will contain xenoestrogens (fake estrogen chemicals) and the bisphenols we talked about earlier. Plastic bottles also contain a leadlike compound called antimony. Your best bet is natural, unprocessed mineral water in glass containers.

Ultraviolet Light

Sunlight contains ultraviolet B waves (UVB). These waves, in moderation, are good for you, for they help the skin make vitamin D_3, the type of vitamin D that is good for mood, immune balance, and cancer protection. But too much UVB is not so good. Like a radioactive substance, it will cause genetic changes, which contribute to both cancer and aging of the skin.

Ultraviolet exposure also accelerates the destructive abilities of a gene called p16, which ages healthy cells much faster than normal. These cells then can't repair themselves, fight off inflammation, or self-replicate. Healthy skin cell replication is a key to beautiful skin.

Too much light at night also suppresses melatonin production, which causes poor sleep. Poor sleep leads to poor ability to clean out toxins, which leads to—you guessed it—aging.

Cell Phones and Electromagnetic Fields (EMFs)

Research shows that holding a cell phone to your head causes increased metabolic activity in areas of the brain closest to the phone. While most people do not develop brain cancer from cell phones, it is thought that for those who have a genetic predisposition, it may be best to limit exposure. I personally use the speakerphone as much as possible, or the headset if people around me are not amenable to a speakerphone (such as on the subway or bus). Electrical wiring also throws off EMFs—and again, we do not know who is susceptible to developing diseases from these.

The Detoxification Process

We learned a lot of scary facts in the previous section. Now here comes the good news: you can do something about all this! Stop the incoming toxins and detoxify to clean your body out.

The following pages will offer you some excellent ways to get your detoxification going. These methods deliver terrific results in my clinic; it's the same rejuvenating program my husband, Peter, and I followed before I started trying to get pregnant. These are the ways to detox, lose weight, arrest your aging, enhance your beauty, and get back energy you may not know you had.

As far as the timing of this detox, you can make each step last as little as one week, or you can take longer for each as needed. No pressure. The important thing is to take your time and follow the steps in order. Just choose a period coming up when things will be relatively quiet: when you don't need to travel, you have time to shop for the foods you'll need— maybe a time that doesn't involve your best friend's wedding.

And be safe. While this detox is very gentle and

nourishing, remember that medications are also processed through the liver. As a result, the levels of the drugs in your system might be affected by a detox. So, if you are taking any medications, check with your prescribing doctor before starting a detoxification regimen.

Detox Step *1*: Stop the Incoming

While I'm not a fan of military analogies, here's one that works to describe how the body can clean itself: When a city is under bombing attack, the citizens generally stay indoors and out of sight. They don't move around, and they certainly do not go outside to throw out the trash. Your body is the same way. It can't effectively clean out the bad if there's still more entering it. There is no way to fix a toxic issue until you have identified where the toxins are coming from and have created a plan to get them out. We've talked about the gerontogens that are aging you prematurely. Now let's get them out of our lives. Here are some cleanup strategies:

Eat Organic, Pesticide-Free, Hormone-Free, Non-GMO Foods

While it is nearly impossible to be 100 percent organic, do your best to purchase organic vegetables and fruits and organic, grass-fed meats. If you need to make financially efficient choices, it's important to know which vegetables and fruits are the most polluted. There are some foods for which you should choose only organic; for others, your choices can be more flexible. Please review "The Essential Organics," in chapter 2. During this detox, the produce that has the distinction of making the dirty list should be more strictly avoided unless it is organic. Apples are a good example. In my home, we eat only organic apples.

GMOs, or genetically modified foods, include injected genetic material not found in the natural world. More than sixty-five countries, including the European Union countries, Australia, and Japan, have pretty much banned these foods. The United States relies on safety testing performed by the very companies that profit from these foods to decide if they are safe for you and me—so in this country, the GMO fox is guarding the henhouse! Not surprisingly, these companies claim that GMOs are safe. Food studies from Europe, however, have shown that GMOs have toxic effects on organ systems and create molecules that push cancer buttons. While not enough studies have definitively proven GMOs to be safe or harmful, my vote is no. Why risk the possible detrimental health effects of GMOs when normal, healthy food is available? The only way to avoid non-GMO foods is to move to a foreign country—or stay in the United States and look for "Non-GMO Project–Verified" foods, a label that means something. And keep telling your legislators (with your wallet and your vote) that you will not stand for GMOs in your food.

If You Smoke, Stop Smoking

Easy to say. Not so easy to do. Some people can simply decide to quit and then stick to that commitment. I applaud them—but that is not the norm. Most people need support to become free from cigarettes. Cigarettes are addictive, and getting off them is not so easy. There are four steps I recommend in my clinic to be smoke-free:

1. Follow the SmokeEnders protocol for seven weeks (www.smokenders.com).

2. During those seven weeks, have regular acupuncture three days a week. There's a set of auricular (outer ear) points that are collectively termed the "five-needle" protocol, which is designed to help with addiction.

3. Eat sunflower seeds; these are known to curb cravings.

4. Also during the seven weeks, start taking Smokeless, a tincture by Wise Woman Herbals. Take five drops when you feel a craving, but don't take more than one hundred drops a day.

Toss Lotions, Antiperspirants, Deodorants, Shampoos, and Perfumes

Get "back to nature" by using natural, toxin-free skin care products, shampoos, and cosmetics. These will revitalize your skin and hair, and help restore your natural beauty. Look at the labels for words such as *parabens* (e.g., *methyl* and *ethyl paraben*), *FDA lake # 5 dye*, *parfum*, and *fragrance*. These are all toxins. Even *natural fragrance* is not natural, so don't fall for it. If you are not sure if a product is clean, check out the Environmental Working Group's website, www.EWG.org.

Clean out the Cleaners

Household cleaning products made from harsh chemicals take a toll on your beauty and increase occurrences of illness and disease. These chemicals take to the air and get into our bloodstreams way too easily. By using safe alternatives, though, you can conserve the energy your body is using to detox and use it to regenerate and revitalize your health and beauty. And since the toxins in most beauty products are harmful to the environment, you will also be conserving the energy and vitality of our earth. A win-win for everyone.

Choose Natural Paints and Textiles

As much as possible, be aware of every chemical that comes into your home or office, and choose the most natural you can. See the box "Common Sources of In-

door Air Pollution." Look for carpets without chemicals, paints with zero volatile oil compounds, and
furniture that does not off-gas.

Common Sources of Indoor Air Pollution

- carpeting
- cleaning products
- craft materials
- drinking water
- dry cleaning
- fireplaces
- garages
- gas stoves
- laundry detergent/fabric softener/dryer sheets
- magazines
- new furniture
- paints
- perfumes
- pesticides
- scented candles
- shoes
- shower water
- tobacco smoke
- upholstery
- water damage

Replace Man-Made Medications
with Natural Remedies

If you are on a medication, ask your doctor if it is absolutely necessary. If you're being prescribed a medication for the first time, challenge your doctor by asking him or her, "If I take two months to try something natural before using this medication, will that put me in any kind of danger?" This will allow your physician to fully defend why you need a specific drug now. If there is no foreseeable impediment to trying the natural route, consider going all natural first. Also think about working with an accredited naturopathic doctor or other holistic physician well trained in seeking the underlying causes of your issue and treating it using more natural means. (See the "Resources" section to find a doc.)

Purchase a High-Quality Water Filter

As we've discussed, most water contains toxins from pipes, polluted water systems, and pharmaceuticals. Also, treated water contains benzenes and chlorine, which are damaging. Protect yourself with a good filter in your kitchen or wherever you get your drinking water. (See the "Resources" section for some high-quality filter choices.)

Purchase High-Quality Air Filters and Add Houseplants

While we cannot do anything immediate about the air outside, we can at least keep the air in our homes and work areas as clean as possible. (Please see the "Resources" section to find an air filter.) If you cannot have air filtration throughout your home, consider keeping one good filter in your bedroom, the place where you do most of your heavy breathing—while you sleep.

The Best Plants to Clear Your Air?

Aloe vera, English ivy, ficus (weeping fig), and spider plants—while these can help remove formaldehyde and benzenes, they are not nearly as effective as a good air filter, so I'd recommend both the plants and the filter. Unfortunately, if you have a mold problem, you may need to ditch the houseplants until the mold is cleared.

Avoid Excessive UVB Radiation

While some sun exposure is healthy, promoting natural vitamin D production, too much will create more oxidation and promote aging in your skin and body.

Also, the use of tanning beds has been shown to be more damaging than moderate sun exposure.

For Best Vitamin D Production

Try not to shower soon after being out in the sun. Wait a few hours to allow the skin to fully convert your natural production of vitamin D.

Turn off the Night-Light

Light in the bedroom is an environmental toxin in itself. A basic rule I give my patients, which I discussed in the section on sleep, is to turn off the bedroom lights and place a hand twelve inches in front of their faces. If they can see their hands, there's too much light in the room. Excess bedroom light has also been shown to increase hormonal imbalances in women.

Choose Low-Mercury Fish*

Even though mercury is now known to be very toxic to the nervous system, it was used commonly in industry and released into the environment. So, today, our oceans are contaminated. Some fish collect mercury more than others. Here's a list to guide you:

---

* Source: Fish Mercury Guide from the National Resources Defense Council (for more info, go to www.gotmercury.org).

Lowest mercury; safe to eat regularly: anchovies, calamari, catfish, caviar, clams, flounder, herring, lobster (spiny and rock), oysters, salmon, sardines, scallops, shrimp, sole, tilapia, trout (freshwater), whitefish.

Lower mercury; eat sparingly: crab, mahimahi, monkfish, snapper, tuna (fresh, albacore, and chunk light).

High mercury; try to avoid: amberjack, bluefish, halibut, Maine lobster, marlin, sea trout, shark, tuna (ahi, bluefin, white albacore).

Avoid Aluminum

Aluminum is found at high levels in our environment. It is toxic to the brain, and research is accumulating that suggests it plays a role in Alzheimer's disease and Parkinson's, too. It may also cause liver toxicity.

Aluminum sources to minimize: aluminum foil, aluminum pots and pans, antacids, antiperspirants, baking powder, bleached flour, buffered aspirin, canned goods, cigarettes and other tobacco products, city drinking water, colloidal mineral supplements, cream of tartar, deodorants, douches, processed cheese, regular table salt. Consider talking to your doctor about minimizing vaccines when possible, or switching out for those without aluminum adjuvant.

Take Your Shoes Off

About 70 percent of chemicals brought into the house come from your shoes. Leave these toxins at the door by not wearing shoes throughout the house. Ask friends and family to do the same when in your home.

House Slippers

My grandmother always made me wear house slippers when I was young. (Their name is funnier when said with a Sicilian accent: "house-ah slippahs.") When I was a kid, I always thought that was weird. Now when I get home, I love taking off my shoes and getting into my house-ah slippahs.

Minimize Cell Phone Use

As I mentioned earlier in this chapter, cell phones emit electromagnetic fields, or EMFs, which can change metabolism in the tissues exposed. There are now clear links to brain cancer, with long-term cell phone use tripling rates. Cell phone use also ups the rates of infertility and can encourage spontaneous abortion. The good news is exposure is worst when you are very close to the phone, so just keeping it a few inches away can help a lot. While I realize it is unrealistic to live without your phone, try these suggestions:

Avoid carrying your cell phone close to your body whenever possible. Leave it in your bag.

When you make a call, use the speakerphone function when you can. When you cannot, use a headset.

Avoid using your phone in moving cars and trains, when signaling EMFs are at their strongest.

Keep babies and kids away from active cell phones. If the kids are playing on them, at least put them on standby or in airplane mode so they're not sending and receiving signals.

In your bedroom, avoid keeping electronic devices near your body and head while sleeping. Many people keep their cell phone on their nightstand. My advice is to keep it on the other side of the room, if possible.

Be Bold and Check the Mold

If you're feeling sick, humidity and mold may be lurking. Mold can set off inflammation in your body and make you sick. I have seen patients with all sorts of health problems due to mold: chronic fatigue, depression, and autoimmune problems, to name a few. Some people are more susceptible than others to this poorly understood health challenge. Testing and treatment require some special work that most doctors are not aware of. (Check the "Resources" section at the end of this book to find a specialist who knows how to test your body and properly treat mold issues.)

Get Political

The only way to rid ourselves of the chemicals in our environment is by urging our local governments to commit to cleaning things up. Please write to your legislators. Be very clear about what you want and don't want. And consider supporting candidates and parties that truly want to change things.

Write to Your Legislators

To locate your federal legislators, visit: www.house.gov/representatives/find/ and www. senate.gov/reference/common/faq/How_to_ contact_senators.htm.

To send a note to your state legislators, visit: openstates.org/find_your_legislator/.

Congratulations, you have made some major strides in minimizing incoming toxins. Now you're ready to start the internal cleaning work.

Detox Step 2: Open the Channels of Detoxification

Eating nutritious food, getting your beauty sleep, meditating, and being physically and mentally active keep your nervous system engaged and interested. These behaviors send signals to every one of your cells to get rid of toxins and stay vital. Vital, well-fed cells communicate with your brain, telling you that you're in good enough shape to have fun and enjoy life.

Let's go over the basics of detoxifying naturally. Please do not skip this second step. Many patients come into my practice after they have done the latest "detox" feeling depleted and worse than before they started. Why? One reason is that they followed a regimen that did not consider how the body works.

For many tasks, preparation is 95 percent of the work. This one is no different. A proper detox starts with "pre-detox," which comprises the basics to opening up the elimination channels. If you don't take these steps, your liver will create more powerful toxins that will have no exit route. (More about liver detoxification in "Fifty Ways to Love Your Liver," under step 3.)

The basics to vital detoxification are:

Sleep

Seven hours of sleep at a minimum, with a regularly scheduled bedtime of no later than 11:00 p.m., is vital for healthy beauty. If getting a restful sleep is a challenge for you, go back to chapter 1 and sort out your sleep situation as best you can. Then come back here.

Good Fluids: Water, Green Tea, and Schizandra

Drink one big glass of purified, room temperature water in the morning and forty to sixty ounces of purified water a day.

Enjoy some green tea in the morning and early afternoon as a sensible and healthy pick-me-up. It not only fights many types of cancers but also supports weight loss and beefs up your antioxidant defenses.

Known in Chinese medicine as wu wei zi, schizandra (the "fruit of five tastes") is one of my all-time favorite teas to support beauty and keep me relaxed. While clearing activated toxins in phase two of liver detox, it supports skin health by protecting your skin from wind and sunburn damage while keeping the mind calm without being a sedative. Drink one cup of this delicious berry tea in the early evening for a calming effect.

Good Food

As just mentioned, foods should be organic and as natural as possible.

> *Protein.* You should consume about 50 g of
> protein a day. Some of my favorite proteins are:
>> Wild salmon;
>> Tilapia (mercury-free)—tilapia has the
>> highest amount of protein of any source
>> available;
>> Grass-fed beef and lamb;
>> Naturally raised poultry;
>> Beans; and
>> Raw nuts and seeds.

Veggies. Eat one cup of cruciferous veggies a day. These include broccoli, bok choy, cauliflower, and Brussels sprouts.

Garlic and onion. Eat these in liberal doses—you may need to check with your partner on this one (at least before smooching!)—as garlic and onion contain sulfur compounds that keep detoxification humming.

Fruit. Eat one organic apple and one cup of organic berries a day. Add a third organic fruit of your choice.

Healthy oils. One tablespoon of extra-virgin organic olive oil every day, packed with skin-supporting omega-9 fats, really is the Italian secret to great skin!

Fiber. There's an old saying: "You have to keep the pipes moving." Well, when it comes to age-making gerontogens and other toxins, if the pipes aren't moving, the body can't get rid of what it needs to. Ideally, you want to consume at least 25 g of fiber in order to rid your body of solid waste at least once a day. If you are not used to getting all that fiber, start slowly; otherwise, you may turn into a very uncomfortable bag o' gas. Here are some ideas to get you "going." Remember, you do not need to add all of these:

> *Dark greens.* Eat one cup a day of cooked dark greens (e.g., kale, chard, dandelion, spinach).

Need a good recipe? Visit www.DrPinaND
.com/greens.

Apples. Eat one apple a day. (Yes, an apple a
day *does* keep the doctor away—in fact, studies
out of both Italy and Poland show that there
was a 50 to 80 percent decrease in many types
of cancers, including prostate, breast, and colon
cancer, when participants ate "one a day.")

Flax meal. One tablespoon of flax meal equals
2 g of fiber, is a great anti–inflammatory, and
helps balance women's hormones.

Organic prunes. Eat two to five prunes a day.
These have astounding antioxidant and
flavonoid content.

Organic celery and carrots. Eat these for an
extra-fibrous crunch. Celery contains 1 g of
fiber per stalk, and one carrot equals about 2 g.
Celery contains 3-n-butylphthalide, which
lowers blood pressure; while carrots have skin-
beautifying lycopene and carotenes.

Lentil or bean soup. Each contains 8 g of fiber
per half cup. Beans have been proven to
prevent breast cancer recurrence by cleansing
the body of excess hormones.

Bowel Besties

Besides eating the right foods, two supplements are a
great help for staying regular every day:

Psyllium. Start with one teaspoon and move slowly up to one or two tablespoons in a big glass of water once a day. Psyllium won't be needed, however, if the fiber foods are working well enough.

Probiotics. These little guys keep the pipes flowing by nourishing and maintaining your intestinal lining. They also help your brain make neurotransmitters so you stay in a good mood. Take eight billion bacteria a day. In my clinic, I recommend a product called Restoraflora (see the "Resources" section at the end of this book): one capsule in the morning and evening.

Extra Bowel-Moving Assistance

Senna and cascara are natural laxatives, but they are habit forming, which means if you take them every day for a long enough time, your body will grow dependent on them. If you are really constipated and need things to move along faster, besides psyllium fiber, you can also add magnesium oxide (500 mg a day) and heaping amounts of vitamin C (2,000 mg three times a day). Magnesium and vitamin C are not habit forming.

Foods to Skip Completely

There are foods that you should not consume during your detox. They are:

> All "white" foods: bread, bagels, pasta, white rice, sugary foods;
>
> All fruit juices. Remember, it's for only a few weeks;
>
> All dairy products (that is, any product made from cow's milk);
>
> All alcohol;
>
> All coffee (green tea is okay);
>
> Any foods with preservatives, added sugars, and any words you can't pronounce or don't understand; and
>
> All fried foods and crispy snacks.

Spirit/Relaxation

Detoxing the body includes detoxing the mind, and intentionally letting go of those things that hold us back. Detoxing can be an important time to:

> *Examine your relationships.* Strengthen the ones that are healthy for you by telling the people who love you that you appreciate and love them, too. This may also be a time to make tough decisions and eliminate relationships with people who don't support you.

Take a break from bad news. Most TV and print news is a series of one negative thought after another (with advertising in between). You don't need it—if it is important, believe me, you'll hear about it. Instead, read books with positivity written all over them. (I've listed a few in the "Resources" section.)

Take a day off from your watch/clock/cell phone. We all live by these devices. Taking a day or two (maybe the weekend?) off helps reset our bodies' natural sense of time.

Exercise

Earlier in the book, we learned that moving your body is an antiaging miracle. This movement is also a key to bona fide detoxification.

❋ Increased circulation brings more flow through the liver and kidneys, which are the main organs of detox. Your lymphatic system is basically the drainage system of your body; it collects waste products and toxins. While the cardiovascular system has a heart to pump the blood around, the lymphatic system has no such built-in pump. Yet every time you move a muscle, your lymphatic system gets a chance to move its contents into the system of veins to help get stuff out. When the muscles do not move, the body cannot detox. If you don't exercise, you will also miss out on sweating, a prime method your body uses to cleanse itself. Also, good deep breathing ensures better cell oxygenation. Finally, exercise removes sub-cutaneous fat, which stores many unwanted toxins.

Dr. Pina's Recommendation for Detox Exercise

Beginners: Thirty minutes of gentle interval aerobic activity four days a week, and two days a week of yoga detoxification poses—perform three sequences (see examples on my website at www.DrPinaND.com/detoxyoga) every four hours for a total of four times a day. Go slowly and hold each pose for five seconds.

Intermediate and advanced: One hour of cardio, with the last thirty minutes including some interval training (exercise that alternates between high and low intensity) four days a week, plus two days of resistance work followed by detoxification yoga—perform three sequences (visit www.DrPinaND.com/detoxyoga for poses) every four hours for a total of four times a day.

Body and mind work: Once a week, do something to balance your energy: massage, acupuncture, or Bikram yoga. You can try Reiki, too.

Detox Step 3: Add Supplements

In step 1 you learned how to stop the incoming. In step 2 you added the basics you needed to clean out things effectively. Now, in step 3, you are going to arm yourself with some supplements known to support the body and clean out the junk.

Fifty Ways to Love Your Liver

The liver is a key to healthy aging. It is the organ responsible for balancing blood sugar, metabolizing hormones, and keeping toxins from staying in the body. We all know how drinking too much alcohol isn't healthy for the liver. And we know that the signs of an unhealthy liver will show up on the skin—in the form of liver spots, excess wrinkles, and an overall unhealthy pale green hue. People with liver problems are easy to spot a mile away. Someone with a healthy liver, however, shines—a healthy liver equals a glowing you.

Topical Help for Hyperpigmentation Spots

Dark patches on the skin, known as hyperpigmentation, are collections of melanin pigment. Niacinamide creams, made with a specific form of vitamin B$_3$ (niacin), help stop melanin pigment from collecting on the skin's surface. In one study, a group of twenty-seven patients with melasma (skin discoloration) was given a 4 percent niacinamide cream on one side of the face and 4 percent hydroquinone on the other. Measurements showed benefits on both sides, with no difference between one side and the other. Since hydroquinone is a fairly toxic, gasoline-like medication, niacinamide may be the better overall choice.

✳ The liver has two phases of detoxification. In phase one, the organ uses the cytochrome system, in which your body takes toxins, chemicals, and drugs and converts them into compounds that are actually even *more* toxic. Don't worry, though—as long as the liver has the right support, it can perform phase two of detoxification. In this phase, these toxic compounds will be ushered from the liver and into the intestines and the bloodstream and taken harmlessly out of the body.

Let's talk about a few of the supplements you can use during your detox to support your liver and make your detoxification really work.

Supplemental protein

I routinely see patients come to me after trying the latest Internet or book cleanse, fast, or detox, and feeling worse than ever. As an example, a very popular cleansing book came out around 2010. Although it was written by a knowledgeable medical doctor, it didn't take into account that to allow for a real detox, the liver (and the body as a whole) needs important support with enough protein. Protein is a vital nutrient that furnishes the amino acids needed for phase two of your detoxification. As a result of trying this low-protein detox, many patients came in to see me not because the cleanse didn't work, but because it only half-worked. It released toxins into their body, but didn't allow those toxins the chance to leave the body. As a result, the patients felt sicker. The cleanse did not support the systems. When your system is not properly supported, it will produce more toxic compounds that can make you feel worse.

Therefore, starting in week three of your detox, take in some extra protein. Take about 30 g a day, in the form of rice protein, pea protein, or hemp.

Cod-liver oil

One teaspoon of a high-quality cod-liver oil supplies you with beautiful omega fats, which are needed to calm inflammation and support great skin, as well as vitamin D and vitamin A. Aim for 5 g (about one teaspoon).

Probiotics

Good bacteria such as *Lactobacillus* and *Bifidus* are key players in helping the body start to detoxify in the intestines, too. Probiotics have been proven to help a toxic body feel better. I recommend a dose of about eight billion twice a day.

Spirulina and chlorella

When the liver starts detoxing, it sends junk into the intestines. A good greens formula will have green chlorella, fiber, and a mix of powdered vegetables. Taken in the morning, it will help to suck up the bad stuff and get it out of the body. In our clinic, for liver-supportive supplements, we use Source Cleanse, cod-liver oil, Restoraflora, and Source Greens. (Please see the "Resources" section to find them.)

Old-time naturopathy: The castor oil pack

The castor oil pack is an age-old naturopathic consti-pation remedy that is still used in some hospitals. It is known to help relax tight muscles, reduce spasms, and gently decrease inflammation while bringing circula-tion to whatever body part it is used on.

Please note that castor oil isn't to drink—it is to place topically over the liver area to support liver de-toxification.

1. Purchase castor oil and an unbleached and undyed flannel from any drugstore or health food store. Unbleached/undyed is best; that way no chlorine or chemical dyes get absorbed into the body.

2. Cut a piece of flannel big enough to cover your liver and abdominal area, then apply a good amount of castor oil over the liver area. The liver is located on your right trunk, between the nipple area and the border of the ribs. If you are constipated or have lots of digestive discomfort, you may want to place the castor oil over the abdomen, using your belly button as a center point.

3. Cover the castor oil with the flannel.

4. Place a heating pad over the flannel, set the temperature to medium (not too hot), and leave it on for up to forty-five minutes. It is pretty relaxing, but please do not go to sleep with the heating pad on.

5. After forty-five minutes, remove the pad. Wash off the castor oil with some soap and water. You can wash the flannel in soapy water, or wrap it in plastic and keep it in the fridge for four more uses; then clean it. Do this every other day, or even every day, for constipation and/or detoxification support.

What About Colonics?

When I was in medical school, we were trained in giving colon hydrotherapy to patients during their detox regimens. I'll be honest—I was not an initial fan of someone sticking a tube in my butt (pardon my language) and cleaning it out with liquid. But as a student clinician, I was amazed to see people leave after the colonic feeling so happy and vital.

Research shows that women who move their bowels well are generally happier, and even have better relationships. (A 2001 research study from the journal *Gut* showed that constipated women found it much harder to form close relationships than unconstipated women.) So a colonic every so often might be beneficial for overall quality of life as well as aid in a detox. Cleaning the colon sends a signal to the liver that it can release more toxins. So a good colonic promotes good liver detoxification.

How Does a Colonic Work?

Colonics entail a professional practitioner inserting a tube into the anus and gently allowing water to flow into the colon, and then stopping the water and allowing the colon to release the water and its contents. This is done a few times per session, and the procedure is usually completed within twenty minutes. While it's not mandatory, I recommend you get a colonic once at the end of each detox week, for the three to five weeks of your detox, but for no more than six weeks.

While generally safe, colonics are not recommended for pregnant women; for people with any bleeding disorder of the intestines, electrolyte imbalance, or ulcerative colitis; or for anyone who is frail. Please speak to your physician to check if a colonic is right for you. (The "Resources" section will help you find a professional practitioner.) There is no official certifying organization for colon therapists, so the best approach is to get a recommendation from your naturopathic doctor or someone you trust.

How Long and How Often to Detox?

....

As mentioned earlier, steps 1 and 2 each take as short as one week. But you can take your time and go longer for each of these if needed. For step 3, I recommend keeping up the regimen for two weeks, if possible. You can go longer if you like. Remember, this is not a fast—so you can eat as much as you want. Just keep it to very healthy eating combined with other lifestyle and supplement choices.

I personally do a regimen like this twice a year, in the spring and fall. These are seasons of change, and ancient medicines such as Chinese medicine suggest that these times of year are a good time for cleaning out and letting go.

Chelation and Advanced Detox Testing

....

You are reading this book to help defy aging and have the healthiest skin possible. The detox steps I've just outlined will help you in your journey toward that goal. Yet there are other, more advanced methods to detox that your health care practitioner can facilitate. One is called chelation. Chelation uses various special compounds to help draw the toxins out of your body.

If you have a history of high toxin exposure (from working with chemicals or living near a highway) and underlying chronic disease, such as autoimmune disease, diabetes, high blood pressure, mood disorder, cardiovascular concerns, difficult rashes, cancer, neurological disorder, or chronic fatigue, you may want to consider advanced detoxification work with your naturopathic physician or other holistic provider to look further into underlying toxicity issues.

With my patients facing these challenging conditions, I recommend special testing, including blood work, urine tests, and hair analysis, to look for the presence of many of the chemicals we mentioned earlier in the chapter, such as heavy metals, PCBs, and POPs. If these toxins show up abnormally in the body, I may recommend specialized chelation or other, more aggressive detoxification work.

For 90-plus percent of my patients, the detox regimen we've just discussed will get the job done for preventive health, antiaging, and enduring beauty and vigor. But if you need extra support and/or have a chronic disease that requires stronger care, chelation is a reasonable next step for you. It should be done under your doctor's supervision, and those with kidney problems or who are very weak may not be able to try this kind of therapy.

Chapter 6

GLOWING SUPPLEMENTS AND HORMONAL HARMONY

I take vitamins.

—HILLARY CLINTON

We have moved through all the food, lifestyle, and thought processes involved in truly getting your best glow. We've detoxed a bit, too. Now comes the easy chapter. It's all about supplements—the vitamins, amino acids, and herbs you can use to achieve your best glow a little faster and a little better than you could without them.

My first recommendation for this chapter is a bit of a gentle warning: if you haven't read the previous chapters and incorporated the diet, lifestyle, and psychological steps that are needed, I can tell you now, despite what the media tells you, there are no "miracle" or "magic bullet" supplements that will make up for that work.

True health and glowing beauty require proper sleep, exercise, relaxation, foods, and lifestyle and supplemental supports all together. Only by cultivating those steps will your body's vitality kick in.

Are Supplements Safe?

The nice thing about using the right supplements with a good naturopathic protocol is not only are you moving toward healing the issue, but the supplements also help get the job done in a much safer way. Many conventional doctors are afraid of herbal medicines because they are supposedly "not well studied" or can have side effects that will mess up other medication's activity.

Yet, in eleven years of practice, I have not seen a single major issue with supplements. If you don't believe me, pore through the research yourself (which I've included in the "References" section at the end of this book). Dr. Arthur Presser is a researcher at the University of Southern California's School of Pharmacy. He has compiled copious information about deaths from herbs, and has found them to be exceedingly rare compared to deaths from conventional medicine (or even typical everyday events). He calculated that there is a 1-in-333 chance of death from properly used medication but only a 1-in-1-million chance of death from the use of herbal remedies.

Herbs and supplements are generally safer because these natural substances talk to your body in ways that processed pharmaceuticals can't. Generally, if you take too much of a vitamin or herb, it will upset your digestion. Manufactured drugs have had processed out of them the natural molecules that talk to the body. For example, Native Americans used the plant foxglove for people with heart issues. If too little was taken, it didn't work. If too much, the person would get nauseated and start vomiting. Medical researchers looked at foxglove and found it contained digitalis, which was made into a drug. Too little digitalis doesn't work, but a little too much will kill you, because it has a strong effect and is devoid of the other plant chemicals that tell your body you are overdosing.

Of course, you need to be smart—just because something is natural, that doesn't mean it's safe. For example, fat-soluble vitamins such as vitamins A and D can be good for certain issues, but when taken at too high a dose, they can also be toxic. Similarly, St. John's wort, which is known to be a phenomenal anxiety and depression buster since the time of Hippocrates, can interfere with many medications, including birth control. When taking herbal supplements, be sure you work with a naturopathic physician or other knowledgeable practitioner, especially if you are taking prescription medication at the same time.

When I make clinical decisions with my patients, I use the wisdom of my teachers, which is based on thousands of years of Native American and Chinese medicine and eclectic herbalism along with rigorous research from the most up-to-date resources we have today. This chapter compiles the best of both worlds to help you live healthier, with more vitality, and find your glow.

The Three Basics

So, what do you take? When you walk into a health food store, it's dazzling and confusing. There is such an array of supplements, such pretty colors and flavors. Which ones to pick? They all look good.

Well, my super-strong suggestion is, before you hop on the latest encapsulated antioxidant superfood bandwagon, start with the tried-and-true basics: a multivitamin, fish oil, and a probiotic.

1. A Good-Quality Multivitamin

My first suggestion is nothing new: it's the good old multiple vitamin, a shotgun approach to nutrition.

"But I eat an excellent diet—I don't need extra vitamins."

You may be saying this to yourself. It makes sense, but it's wrong. Why? Because it has been shown that even those eating a healthy diet are often deficient in vitamins and minerals. In 2006 the *Journal of the Inter-*

national Society of Sports Nutrition published a review analysis of seventy different diets and found that none of them, even the healthiest ones, reached the full recommended daily amount of the basic vitamins and minerals. For athletes and exercisers, the nutrient levels were even lower because these people were burning through more.

I totally agree that food is by far the best source of nutrients. In a perfect world of soils that are fertilized well with organic compost and farms that do not use pesticides, a good balanced diet would get the job done. Unfortunately, the research is clear that today's food, grown in soils greatly deficient in the vitamins and minerals they contained fifty years ago, are not producing the nutrients they used to. This has been well studied. In 2004 an important study out of the University of Texas compared the nutrient data of forty-three veggies and fruits in the years 1950 and 1999. Published in the *Journal of the American College of Nutrition*, the study found significant decreases in basic food nutrition. Other work, from the Kushi Institute, found drops of up to 40 percent in levels of calcium, iron, and vitamin C. According to *Scientific American*, you would have to eat eight oranges to get the same amount of vitamin A that our grandparents would have enjoyed from only one! Vitamin A is important for protecting the lining of our respiratory tract—no wonder we seem to get sick more often. (I thought it was the lack of sleep.)

Did you know that a year 2000 Women's Health

Study performed at Emory University looked at more than 4,500 women physicians and found that female docs take multiple vitamins as much as or more often than the general population? They are pretty smart ladies—and they know about the research I am going to share with you now.

Remember when we talked about telomeres protecting our DNA and reducing aging? (If you don't, see the previous chapter.) Telomeres are associated with greater health and possibly longer life. Well, a 2009 study in *The American Journal of Clinical Nutrition* looked at 586 women aged thirty-five to seventy and found more than a 5 percent increase in telomere length in those who took a daily multivitamin. That's pretty impressive, since telomeres usually tend to get shorter as we age, not longer.

In another study, done in 2011, researchers out of Australia gave fifty healthy men (aged fifty to seventy) either a multiple vitamin or a placebo. They found that the men who took the real vitamin felt less stressed out and had less depression and more energy—and they were able to be more productive. And in Sweden, the Stockholm Heart Epidemiology Program from the early 2000s found that a low-dose multivitamin supplement may aid in the primary prevention of heart attack in both men and women. A newer, 2015 study of more than 8,600 people found a 35 percent decrease in death from heart problems among women who took a multiple vitamin for more than three years.

B Vitamins for Skin and Nails

Brown-gray nails? Take vitamin B_{12}.
Lip corner dryness? Take vitamin B_2 (riboflavin).
Nail ridging? Try the methylfolate form of folic acid.

Should I Take a Supplement with Iron?

Unless their blood has tested high for iron, most pre-menopausal women should take an iron supplement. Postmenopausal women (and men) should not take an iron supplement unless they are low in iron and medical reasons for this have been ruled out.

Capsules or Tablets?

If you are buying an over-the-counter vitamin, look for a capsule (not a tablet; tablets are usually cheaply made and contain binders you don't want). Also, look for a vitamin with good manufacturing practices (GMP) certification.

Is More Better?

I don't recommend high-dosing vitamins in general. Just because they are good for you, it doesn't mean taking more is better. In nature, you generally don't get tons of vitamins at one time, so take the prescribed amount of a good-quality multiple, and see a naturo-pathic doctor before deciding to high-dose a vitamin.

With Food or Without?

Multiple vitamins should always be taken with food, since some of the vitamins in multivitamins (such as A, D, E, and K) are best absorbed with food. Also, if not taken with food, minerals such as zinc can cause some people nausea or bellyaches.

What Happens If I Skip a Dose?

I take my multiple vitamin five or six days a week, so I skip one day every week. It's fine to take a little time off with your vitamins. They are not drugs, you know.

2. Fish Oil

Where do I begin when touting the benefits of fish oil? We've talked a little bit about the central role of fish oil in the Mediterranean diet. Now we are going to talk about why fish oil supplementation every day (or most days) will work to build your glow.

✳ Fish oil has two main components, eicosapen-taenoic acid (EPA) and docosahexaenoic acid (DHA), which are also important components of every cell membrane in your body. Cell membranes are responsi-ble for bringing nutrients in and carting the junk out, and for a balanced and appropriate immune reaction (one that isn't too weak, as in immune deficiency, or too strong, as in autoimmune or allergic reactions). Finally, cell membranes help create communication among cells. When cells don't communicate well, the body gets sick. People who have a regular intake of fish oil have happier moods, less anxiety, and greater overall health.

Ohio State University College of Nursing studies describe how fish oil supplementation has also been shown to help lower inflammation and increase the benefits of your body's wound-healing mechanisms. In people who took fish oil supplements, wounds were shown to heal faster and with less scarring than in people who did not take fish oil. Other studies show that those who take fish oil have less skin sensitivity and fewer breakout rashes from ultraviolet sunlight exposure.

Dosage

I generally recommend about 1,000 mg of EPA per dose of fish oil. Read the label carefully. If it does not list the actual EPA content, then buy a fish oil that does. Also, your fish oil should be in "triglyceride form" and "molecularly distilled." Molecular distillation is a process that removes contaminants such as mercury and PCBs. If your fish oil does not ensure this, stay away from it. I prefer taking cod-liver oil (about one teaspoon a day), for it also has a little extra vitamin D and A. Especially moving into the fall and winter, that extra D and A will help ward off the flu.

Fish oil can be taken as a gelcap or liquid. Liquid fish oil should be kept in the refrigerator after opening. If you have stomach trouble and you find that fish oil makes you burp or gives you reflux, look for an enteric-coated version, which will not cause discomfort.

Oils for Vegans?

While vegan oils such as flax and sesame oil may have some benefits, they need to be converted to EPA in the body. Unfortunately for many people who are not healthy, the enzyme used to do this is often not functioning well. As a result, these oils may not fully support your system the way fish oil can. If it is not possible for you to take fish oil for ethical reasons or because of an allergy, you might consider algae-derived essential fats, flax oil, or rapeseed oil. The best sources of vegan omega-3 fats are found in these oils; you can get some also in walnuts and tofu.

3. Probiotics

Probiotics are the third in my triumvirate of favorite supplements. Probiotics are the good germs that line our digestive tract by the billions. As a group, they are called the microbiome, which is a hot topic in medical research right now. It turns out there are ten times more of them than there are cells in our bodies! So, do you think probiotics are important? I do.

These little cuties were originally studied in the 1800s, by Russian bacteriologist Elie Metchnikoff, who realized that people could enhance their health and delay their cognitive decline by eating yogurt to improve the microbiome. As often happens in medicine, one researcher's good work and selfless pursuit of healthy information was virtually ignored until relatively recently.

How to Live to a Hundred

Russian researcher Elie Metchnikoff described the people who lived to the healthy age of one hundred (and this was one hundred years ago—*before* antibiotics and good sanitation) as "poor or of humble circumstances, with extremely simple life styles."

This led him to recommend being "moderate in food and drink and in all other pleasures," complemented by daily exercise "whatever be the weather . . . lived in a peaceful environment in which the air is pure . . . going to bed early and rising early after not more than 6–7h of sleep, bathing daily with water neither too hot nor too cold, engaging in regular work and mental stimulation, and avoiding alcohol, other stimulants and narcotics."

Sounds like a great, solid naturopathic plan to me!

Today, the National Institutes of Health has a well-funded Human Microbiome Project, and even a peer-reviewed journal exclusively devoted to the microbiome. I hope that laboratory has a big portrait of Metchnikoff hanging on the wall, in homage to a researcher way ahead of his time.

For years, probiotics have been well known for supporting digestive health and reducing problems associated with infectious diarrhea. As with fish oil, supplementation with probiotics has also been shown to balance immune reaction and support great mood.

Bad Mood? Take Your Probiotics

Lactobacillus and *Bifidobacterium* probiotics were administered for one month and were shown to lower psychological distress and depression and improve problem solving in participants, when compared with a placebo group. Probiotics also increase the relaxing brain neurotransmitter gamma-aminobutyric acid (GABA, which we discussed in chapter 1). As a result, they also helped decrease anger and hostility, while lessening anxiety. You may want to slip some powdered probiotics into your boss's coffee!

Dosage

I recommend using a *Lactobacillus-Bifidus* combination. While there are many other strains out there, and more research needs to be done, these two are backed by the strongest research. Depending on the patient, I prescribe a dosage of about eight billion a day. If a patient is taking antibiotics, I will double the probiotic dose. If you buy an over-the-counter version, don't be cheap. When I was in medical school, one of my teachers found that most of the over-the-counter versions did not contain the strains they were supposed to, and some actually had dangerous bugs such as *E. coli* (which causes food poisoning). Other studies, by ConsumerLab, have seen similar issues.

For multivitamins, fish oil, and probiotics, in our clinic, and for my family, I use the supplements found at www.3UNeed.com. (More about these can be found in the "Resources" section.)

Other Supplements for Your Best Glow

For outer glow as well as inner beauty and health, I have a few other favorite supplements for you to keep in mind.

Vitamin D

Over the past decade, tremendous public interest has accompanied research on vitamin D. Vitamin D is actually a hormone and is responsible not only for good bone health but also for immune system balance, cardiovascular health, cancer protection, and positive mood. It's obtained most easily from the sun, but the modern world we live in is constantly blocking out sun. Clothes, vehicles, buildings, and even pollution will stop the ultraviolet light from reaching our skin to produce the D we need. Whether it is accidental or by design, most of us are not getting enough sunlight. As a result, people's vitamin D levels are plummeting. In fact, it has been estimated that shunning the sun may prevent skin cancer, but at the cost of allowing fifty-five other cancers to flourish due to low amounts of vitamin D. Vitamin D supplementation provides skin cancer protection and skin-protective effects.

What Is the Safest Sunblock?

While there are many sunblocks out there, I usually use one made with zinc oxide. In this way I avoid exposure to high-toxicity chemicals such as oxybenzone and homosalate, which are found in most over-the-counter sunscreens. Zinc oxide is capable of reflecting a broad spectrum of both UVA and UVB rays. It does not penetrate the skin, and has low potential for toxic or allergic effects. Rub onto skin a half hour before going in the sun.

Dosage

There are two types of D on the market: D_2 and D_3. Plants manufacture vitamin D_2, whereas vitamin D_3 is synthesized by humans in the skin when it is exposed to UVB rays from sunlight. In the clinic, I tend to use vitamin D_3, which has been studied the most. I recommend getting your vitamin D level tested. If it's low (under 30 or 40), start taking 1,000 to 2,000 IU of vitamin D_3 with food every day. Recheck in three months. If your D level is still not going up, then you may need to double the dose and recheck in another three months. While typically not enough to raise levels to optimal, the best dietary source of vitamin D is fish. Also, eggs, mushrooms, butter, and parsley have small amounts of D.

Supplements for Hair, Skin, and Nails

What follows are a few of my favorite skin, hair, and nail nutrients. I have used them myself and recommend them to scores of happy ladies. Each is quite safe, and can be very effective when used with the naturopathic program in this book.

Wrinkles? Try GTF Chromium

GTF stands for glucose tolerance factor, a complex molecule that contains the mineral chromium. GTF chromium is found naturally in the body and works by balancing blood sugar. As you'll recall, blood sugar crystals are involved in making advanced glycation end products (AGEs), which are a major player in the aging of your tissues—they age your body the way air makes bread crusty. The more AGEs you have, the more you get crusty and age. (We discussed AGEs in chapter 2.) GTF chromium helps insulin work its best and may aid in fighting wrinkles by controlling blood sugar. It helps control the sugar spikes that can damage the vessels that keep your skin looking young and vital. (Visit www.DrPinaND.com to link to a video of me discussing this nutrient on *The Dr. Oz Show.*)

Dosage

An optimal dose of GTF chromium is 200 mcg twice a day with your food.

Varicose Veins? Try Hesperidin

Veins are the vessels in our body that carry blood away from tissues and back to the heart and lungs. Varicose veins—usually dark purple, wormlike bumps under skin—show up when this natural piping loses its strength and gets out of shape. While genetics can play a role in how prominent varicose veins become as we age, we also know that obesity, excessive constipation, and poor nutrition can play a role.

Hesperidin is a bioflavonoid found in citrus fruits such as lemons and oranges, particularly in the peel and the white stringy area. (The parts of whole fruits we tend to throw away are chock-full of this bioflavonoid.) Bioflavonoids are natural plant pigments with amazing health-giving properties. Flavonoids are the phytonutrients a plant makes to protect itself from ultraviolet radiation, pests, and stress. Taking in flavonoids can help you, too. Hesperidin helps your veins by increasing venous tone, or tightness, and reducing stasis, which is the pooling of poorly moving blood in the veins. It also seems to lower inflammation in veins.

Dosage

To work most effectively, hesperidin should be taken in one 50 mg dose per day. It seems to work even more effectively in combination with another flavonoid, called diosmin, which can be dosed at 450 mg a day. One study looked at more than five thousand people with problems such as varicose veins and found that those who took hesperidin and diosmin for six months saw clear improvement. Food sources of this bioflavonoid include oranges, lemons, tangerines, and grapefruit. You would have to eat about two tablespoons of peel to get a reasonable dose for therapeutic use. A 16-ounce glass of orange juice has about 300 mg of hesperidin—but this has almost 40 g of sugar, so I don't recommend juice as a regular source.

While hesperidin may not completely get rid of varicose veins that are already well established, it may help stop them from growing larger and will prevent others from showing up.

Even Safe in Pregnancy

According to a study published in the *International Journal of Gynecology and Obstetrics*, hesperidin and diosmin were even safe and effective during pregnancy—a time when women tend to get varicose veins and hemorrhoids from the weight of the baby putting pressure on the veins.

Weak and Thinning Hair? Try Black Currant

Black currant fruits and juice, commonly consumed in many parts of the world, are known to be rich in a flavonoid called anthocyanoside, and also contain gamma linolenic acid (GLA). GLA can help balance hormones, strengthen cell membranes, and lower inflammation. These currants and their GLA can help ease eczema, rheumatoid arthritis, premenstrual syndrome, and attention-deficit disorder. GLA helps strengthen hair: it decreases breakage by preventing the hormonal imbalances that weaken and thin your hair.

Dosage

A typical supplemental dose of black currant is 500 mg twice a day. You can also eat black currants, but the supplement oil is made from its seeds, so it would be difficult to achieve the same dosage with only the food.

Want Better-Looking Skin? Try Pycnogenol

Pycnogenol is a bioflavonoid-rich supplement that supports glowing, beautiful skin, aids cardiovascular health, and reduces inflammation. It may be my all-time-favorite supplement for overall glow.

Also called French maritime pine bark extract, this supplement is sourced near the Bordeaux region of France (an area best known for amazing wine), in a forest where pesticides and herbicides are not allowed. The tree bark itself is harvested after twenty-five to thirty years, once the flavonoids have grown to their full level. The use of this flavonoid dates back more than two thousand years, to the time of Hippocrates, and was also used for wounds and ulcers by Native Americans.

✳ Pycnogenol flavonoids are super antioxidants and increase your cells' antioxidant capabilities up to two times. These wonderful bioflavonoids also support your blood vessels and minimize the effects of stress on your heart and vascular system.

How does pycnogenol work?

Decreases AGEs

As we've discussed a few times in this book, a major reason we get wrinkles is the production of advanced glycation end products (known appropriately as AGEs).

Research shows that the flavonoids in pycnogenol can attach to components of our skin called collagen and elastin and protect these from being broken down by excess AGEs. Collagen and elastin are important for keeping skin structure healthy and looking young. When pycnogenol binds with collagen and elastin it helps rebuild elasticity, which is essential for a smooth, younger look.

Aids Skin Circulation

Because pycnogenol is good for the blood vessels, it also helps the micro–blood vessels in the skin stay healthy, which brings better oxygen and nutrient supply to the skin. Supporting the vessels aids in removing toxins and the buildup of metabolic by-products that can normally sit in the skin and make it look older. By improving microcirculation, pycnogenol can help reduce under-eye puffiness caused by leaky capillaries.

Protects Skin from the Sun's Rays

Plant flavonoids naturally protect the plant from the harmful rays of the sun so that the seeds are not dried up and destroyed by ultraviolet radiation. Pycnogenol also defends human skin against the free radicals produced by UV rays, stress, and environmental damage.

Got Melasma?

Some studies also show pycnogenol's benefit in treating melasma, a skin condition of overpigmentation commonly found on the cheeks of women suffering from hormonal imbalance and after pregnancy.

Aids Elasticity and Water Composition

Pycnogenol also stimulates the production of collagen and hyaluronic acid, which enable better skin elasticity and water retention. Without hyaluronic acid and collagen, the skin does not hold water as well and looks thinner, more wrinkled, and not as glowing or vital.

Supports Other Systems

Pycnogenol also decreases the symptoms of asthma and allergies by reducing inflammation. It is well known in the natural medicine world to help the cardiovascular system by supporting blood vessels in artery disease and chronic venous insufficiency. Double-blind trials have proven that pycnogenol helps lower blood pressure, can normalize poor clotting function and cognitive decline from aging, prevents swelling (edema), and may even be useful in attention issues such as attention-deficit and hyperactivity disorder (ADHD). Pycnogenol may also improve the hot flash and night sweat symptoms of menopause.

Dosage

Most studies recommend 50 mg one to three times a day. Some studies suggest 100 mg three times a day. Pycnogenol can be taken with or without food. I use the pycnogenol put out by Douglas Laboratories.

Reaction to Sunlight? Try Polypodium Leucotomos

Used for more than twenty years in Europe, *Polypodium* does a great deal. Like the healthy foods high in antioxidant content we discussed in chapter 2, this strangely named herb will help block the negative effects of ultraviolet rays on your skin's DNA while mopping up the extra free radicals and oxidants that are being produced for up to two hours after ingestion. Solid research suggests it can reduce the number of cells that get burned by the sun.

Dosage

Take 200 mg of *Polypodium leucotomos* as a leaf extract once a day. If you are going outside, take it about forty-five minutes before exposing yourself to the sun. No toxic effects are known when it is given to adults; more studies are welcome to find out if it can be used safely with children and taken over the longer term. Since other types of fern plants may interact with blood pressure and heart medications, check with your prescribing doctor if you plan on trying *Polypodium*.

Recommended Antioxidants

··

Vitamin C and Vitamin E

Known to be taken together, vitamin C (ascorbic acid) and vitamin E (tocopherol) can help jump-start your antioxidant processes. Deficiency of vitamin C will cause skin fragility, irregular bleeding into the skin (in spots known as petechiae), and slow healing of wounds. Vitamin E helps prevent the stiffening of skin due to collagen "cross-linking" (in which collagen fibers stick together). It also helps reduce the oxidation of fats in the blood, called lipid peroxidation. Vitamin E is best taken as a mixed-tocopherol complex, which is a collection of various vitamin E compounds. This is how vitamin E appears in nature. Vitamin C helps regenerate vitamin E. Studies show that using these together is more protective than using them individually.

Dosage

I recommend 500 mg of vitamin C three times a day, and 400 IU of mixed-tocopherol vitamin E. You can find vitamin C in higher amounts in citrus fruits, kiwi, black currants, parsley, rose hips, guavas, and chili peppers (if you can stand the heat). Good natural sources of vitamin E include corn, wheat germ oil, sunflower oil, and safflower oil.

Carotenes
Beta-Carotenes, Astaxanthin, and Lycopene

Your skin holds on to carotenoids close to the surface to protect itself. All related to vitamin A, these beautiful antioxidants have also been shown to protect our mitochondria from DNA damage after being exposed to radiation. That's great, because mitochondrial DNA is not very well protected. As discussed in chapter 5, when the mitochondria break down, we lose an important basic energy supplier, and our chances of disease, especially neurologic diseases and diabetes, go way up.

❋ In one study, people supplemented 25 mg of beta-carotene with some vitamin E for twelve weeks before being exposed to ultraviolet light. The people who took the carotenes showed clear decreases in their propensity to get rashy and red. A trial studying women looked at using 4 mg of astaxanthin per day and found it helped reduce fine lines and wrinkles while improving skin elasticity. Higher doses of 6 mg were beneficial to men. Other studies of astaxanthin show benefits for athletic performance and reduction in stomach inflammation.

Dosage

Beta-carotene is commonly dosed at 25,000 IU with food once a day. Lycopene has been shown to be protective against the sun when the natural extract is taken in a 6 mg dose before sun exposure. For astaxanthin, common dosing is 4 mg once or twice a day. Some studies suggest that for maximum protection, it is best to take these skin-protective supplements for a few weeks. Because high doses of vitamin A should be avoided during pregnancy, pregnant women should speak to their physician before taking these natural carotenes.

Food Sources

If you are looking for more carotenes, probably the best way to get them into your system and take advantage of all the benefits they provide is by eating pumpkin, sweet potatoes, mangoes, papaya, and of course carrots. Astaxanthin is found in algae, yeast, salmon, trout, shrimp, and shellfish. Lycopene is found in many naturally red foods such as tomatoes and watermelon. (Surprisingly, it is missing from cherries and strawberries.)

Recommended Polyphenols

We talked a little about phenols when discussing Rachael Ray's EVOO in chapter 2. Phenols comprise a group of various compounds that belong to the same family as flavonoids. Because they can't protect themselves from danger in nature by running away, the way animals can, plants produce phenol compounds, which give them physical strength so they don't get chewed up and protect them against ultraviolet radiation so they don't burn up. When we ingest them, these compounds confer protection to us, too. Found in green tea and berries and grapes, phenols get broken down when heated to very high temperatures, another reason (besides your food's AGE content) to cook your food at a lower temperature.

Green Tea

Green tea was used first by meditative monks looking to attain calm wakefulness. Green tea is calming due to theanine, an amino acid known to help increase more meditative levels of consciousness. Theanine can also lower blood pressure. Of course, the gentle caffeine content (about a quarter that of coffee) will help keep you more alert and awake. So green tea is perfect if you want to meditate but don't want to fall asleep doing it.

Green tea also contains epigallocatechin-3-gallate (EGCG), which is known for its powerful cancer-fighting and gene-protecting effects (called methylation). This powerful antioxidant has been shown to help keep animal skin cells from turning cancerous in the presence of powerful ultraviolet light. One skin-aging study looked at forty women who, for eight weeks, were given either a combination regimen of topical 10 percent green tea cream and 300 mg twice-daily green tea oral supplementation or a placebo regimen. While the study wasn't long enough to see visual changes, when the researchers looked at the skin cells under a microscope, they found that the people using the cream and supplement did have significant improvement in skin elasticity.

Dosage

Most studies from Japan suggest six cups of tea a day for optimal results (which is three American cups, as our dishes and plates are bigger). You can also take a green tea extract supplement if you prefer.

Is Black Tea as Good as Green Tea for My Skin?

You might be surprised to learn that green and black tea come from the same plant, *Camellia sinensis*. The difference is in leaf preparation: green tea leaves are steamed and then dried; the leaves for black tea are allowed to oxidize. While black tea does have some health benefits, the polyphenol and EGCG content is higher in green tea. Therefore, green tea tends to be healthier overall, and better for the skin.

Pterostilbene

Pterostilbene hails from the modest blueberry and acts as its antioxidant. It's a cousin of the more well-known resveratrol, found in red wine. Studies have shown its benefits in lowering blood sugar, protecting your brain from Alzheimer's, and protecting against cancer, blood disorders, and nervous system diseases all at the same time. It does this likely by protecting your body's cells from the progressive cellular damage and functional problems that come with aging and disease.

✳ Pterostilbene acts through a gene receptor called the peroxisome proliferator-activated receptors (PPARs for short—but don't worry; there won't be a quiz). These receptors help decide whether genes get turned on or off. Like much in natural medicine, this works by an epigenetic mechanism, like the ones we talked about in the introduction.

Dosage

Current studies of pterostilbene have looked at dosages from 100 mg to 450 mg without finding side effects. I recommend 100 mg a day. More studies are needed to understand the benefits, but so far, clinical studies are showing some impressive ones, including lowering of high blood sugar markers and reduction in unhealthy lipids, with no toxicity.

Aloe Vera

The word *Aloe vera* translates from an Arabic word meaning "shining bitter substance" and the Latin word for "true." My aunt Maria was a woman ahead of her time. As a kid, I remember whenever there was a health concern, she'd recommend aloe. That's where I first heard of using it medicinally. While most of us think of it as a salve for burns, even Greeks thought of it as a panacea for many health ills. The Greeks' (and Aunt Maria's) intuition is now well supported by more and more research.

A 2012 Korean study looked at the crow's feet and skin elasticity levels of thirty women of an average age of fifty-six. They gave the women about a quarter teaspoon (not much) of aloe gel by mouth every day for three months and checked their skin again. The researchers found incredible results: the skin wrinkling and roughness had decreased and elasticity had improved.

Research from the 1990s suggests that aloe leaf can contribute to colon cancer. Most aloe preparations sold for ingestion, however, are sold as gel, which is from *inside* the fleshy leaf (called the "inner fillet"). You should never eat the outer part of the leaf, which contains latex and aloin A (both laxative-like compounds). It is irritative to the bowel and can push colon cancer buttons.

Topical Aloe

When aloe is applied topically, it helps the skin produce an antioxidant protein called metallothionein, which helps the body round up the loose oxidants that are causing damage. Kind of like a cowboy roping in wild horses before they destroy the barn.

Dosage

If you plan on taking aloe to support your skin, take only what you need (a small dose of a quarter teaspoon once a day), and make sure it is only the inside, gel part and not the whole leaf. If you have a family history of colon cancer, or are at risk for it, you may want to skip this recommendation, to be extra cautious.

Can Supplements Substitute for Drugs?

....

While supplements are very supportive to the body, you should never just stop medication and take a supplement. That can be dangerous. My clinical experience tells me that natural medicines are beneficial in supporting the body and helping you get to a place of greater health that may allow you to wean yourself off medications with your prescribing doctor's okay. To do this, however, you should be working with a qualified naturopathic physician or other integrative practitioner. Remember, as helpful as they are, supplements are not drug substitutes, so if you are using medication for a life-threatening condition, you should always continue that medication, and consult your prescribing doc about trying natural options.

For example, when someone has shoulder pain or frozen shoulder, which often happens to overworked, stressed-out women in their fifties, the patient is given anti-inflammatory drugs. The drugs stop pain by shutting down the immune system in the area. Sometimes this is accomplished by shooting corticosteroids into the joint. That, indeed, will stop the pain, but it isn't fixing the problem. In fact, it's been shown that when you consistently use anti-inflammatories, the joint problem gets worse because these drugs also stop circulation to the area.

In the naturopathic world, we would use massage and acupuncture, along with contrast hot-and-cold hydrotherapy (see www.DrPinaND.com/contrast for more information) to stimulate the body to bring healing and relief. If you're experiencing shoulder pain, you might need to deal with stress to help relax those tight muscles. Along with this lifestyle work, consider using the right supplements: possibly glucosamine (which helps support joint cartilage repair) and herbs such as curcumin and bromelain (to relieve the pain by balancing immune function—not suppressing it). In this context, supplements and herbs can do their best work. I have seen natural regimens such as these help not only musculoskeletal issues but also problems related to the autoimmune system, digestion, blood pressure, and menopause. The key is to approach these things safely and smartly.

The following table shows what your options are for increasing your glow with supplements. Please remember, you don't have to take all these! Start with

Supplemental Summary

Glow Supplement Supporter	Dose and Directions	Use for
Multiple vitamin	Follow package instructions. Take with food.	General overall health and vitality
Fish oil	Take 1,000 mg EPA per dose per day.	General health and skin health/good for balancing inflammation
Probiotics (*Lactobacillus* and *Bifidus*)	Take 8 billion twice a day.	General health/ digestive health
Vitamin D$_3$	Common dosage is 1,000 IU to 5,000 IU a day. Take with fats for better absorption.	Vitamin D deficiency. Helps mood, skin, digestive function, cardiovascular system, bones, and much more.
GTF chromium	Take 200 mcg once or twice a day with food.	Blood sugar imbalances (prediabetes or diabetes) and if you get "hangry" (hungry + angry)
Hesperidin and diosmin	Take 50 mg hesperidin and 450 mg diosmin a day.	Varicose veins, hemorrhoids
Black currant oil	Take 500 mg a day.	Weak and thinning hair
Pycnogenol	Take 50 mg one to three times a day.	Aging and wrinkled skin, stiffening skin, puffy eyes

Reactions/Side Effects	Best Food Sources
None	Healthy food: green veggies and fruits
Talk to your doctor before using if you're on drugs that affect clotting. You can take an "enteric-coated" version if you have reflux. Don't take if you are allergic to fish.	Fish (surprise!)
None. Check with your doctor if you're having any digestive bleeding.	Yogurt, kimchi, natto, miso, sauerkraut, and other fermented foods
Monitor with laboratory tests, as vitamin D toxicity can cause heart issues due to changes in blood calcium levels.	Along with getting sunlight on the skin, eat fish, eggs, parsley, mushrooms, and butter.
None. Monitor blood sugar if you're taking blood sugar medications.	Brewer's yeast
None. Safe even during pregnancy.	Citrus fruits such as oranges and lemons
None known	Black currants
None known	None

Supplemental Summary

Glow Supplement Supporter	Dose and Directions	Use for
Polypodium leucotomos	Take 200 mg once a day, or forty-five minutes prior to sun exposure—best taken for a few weeks to achieve full effect.	Reactivity to the sun
Vitamin C and vitamin E	Take 500 mg of vitamin C three times a day and 400 IU of mixed-tocopherol vitamin E a day. Vitamin E should be taken with food.	Skin fragility, slow healing, and skin stiffness
Beta-carotenes, astaxanthin, and lycopene	Beta-carotenes: 25 mg a day. Astaxanthin: 4 mg to 6 mg a day. Lycopene: 6 mg a day. Take these three for a few weeks for best effect.	If you easily turn rashy in the sun; for fine lines and wrinkles
Green tea	Drink three cups a day, or take a high-quality green tea extract.	Low mood, cancer prevention, skin health, and much more
Pterostilbene	Take 100 mg a day.	Aging associated with cholesterol and high blood sugar/diabetes
Aloe vera	Take ¼ teaspoon of the gel (inner fillet) orally.	Crow's feet, poor skin elasticity, digestive issues, and skin inflammation

Reactions/Side Effects	Best Food Sources
None known	None
Too much vitamin C can cause loose stools. Don't take more than 800 IU vitamin E per day.	Vitamin C: citrus fruits, kiwi, black currants, parsley, rose hips, guavas, and chili peppers. Vitamin E: corn, wheat germ oil, sunflower oil, and safflower oil.
None known at given doses	Carotenes: pumpkin, sweet potatoes, mangoes, and papaya. Astaxanthin: algae, yeast, salmon, trout, shrimp, and shellfish. Lycopene: naturally red foods (e.g., tomatoes and watermelon).
May cause sleeplessness or anxiety if you are sensitive to caffeine	Green tea
None known at recommended dosage	Blueberries and grapes
Safe. Certain preparations associated with colon cancer (see page 185 for explanation).	Inner fillet of aloe plant

the basic three, and then pick the one or two supplements that seem most suited to your needs.

Hormonal Harmony

....

Whoever thought up the word mammogram? *Every time I hear it, I think I'm supposed to put my breast in an envelope and send it to someone.*

—JAN KING, AUTHOR, BREAST CANCER SURVIVOR,
AND HUMORIST

Many of you might be thinking, "Hey, I'm not in my twenties anymore. I need to get me some of those hormones to stop aging so fast and reduce my wrinkles."

Well, it is true that by age thirty, many hormone levels start dropping. The main estrogens we think about for women are estrogen and progesterone. Estrogen is the yin to progesterone's yang. It is the primary female hormone that helps sex drive and gives us the attributes we think about as womanly (such as lush hair, healthy-looking sex organs, and soft skin). Progesterone is a calming, relaxing hormone that balances estrogen so it doesn't dominate. When estrogen is relatively strong, it can cause headaches, painful and heavy periods, as well as sleep problems. Progesterone also balances your thyroid, keeps you warmer (the reason pregnant women are like a furnace), and helps you let go of fluid you don't need. The research on natural progesterone in women shows that it helps calm the brain, improve sleep, and even raise libido. Progesterone greatly decreases when you are stressed out, because the body naturally shifts to making stress hormones such as cortisol instead. Think about it: in the world of nature, an animal that is constantly running from a bear is not going to be thinking about having sex. While most humans are not running from bears these days, the stress of work, taking care of kids, making ends meet, worrying about elderly parents, and rushing from here to there can send very similar signals to our primitive brain as if there were a bear coming at us. This will cause your body to shunt your hormones away from making proper amounts of progesterone.

Typically, by the time a woman reaches her late thirties, her progesterone starts to flag a bit (sometimes contributing to insomnia, a little more anxiety, and reduced fertility). Then, by the mid- to late forties, her estrogen starts to get imbalanced, contributing to fun menopausal symptoms such as low libido, weight gain, hot flashes, and of course wrinkles. Many women feel this is when they lose their glow.

During the monthlong menstrual cycle, a woman notices changes in her skin: it is thinner at the start of the menstrual cycle, when estrogen and progesterone levels are low, and then it thickens up with the rising levels of estrogen. That lowering of estrogen in the forties and beyond also makes your skin less taut, less able to heal, more wrinkled, drier, and less firm. In postmenopause, skin thickness decreases 1 percent a year, and collagen decreases 2 percent a year.

Hormone Replacement Therapy Versus Natural Hormones

No question: Hormone replacement therapy (HRT) and topically applied estrogen have been shown to increase hydration and blood flow in the epidermis (that top layer of skin), increase skin elasticity and thickness, reduce skin wrinkling, and support the content and quality of collagen. It also protects against the aging effects of the sun.

In the 1960s, it was thought that estrogen and HRT would be miracle cures for women: they would reduce menopausal symptoms; plus they would protect the bones and the heart at the same time. While conventional medicine claimed this issue had been well studied, up until the late 1990s no one had really tested these synthetic hormones. Then, in 2002, a very large study known as the Women's Health Initiative showed that Prempro (a combination of synthetic estrogens made from horse urine plus synthetic progesterone known as medroxyprogesterone acetate) increased heart disease rates, stroke, and blood clots. As if that weren't terrifying enough, these synthetic hormones were also shown to increase breast and ovarian cancer rates. Modern medicine's big "oops" revealed that there were fourteen thousand extra breast cancers a year due to these synthetic hormones—and it seemed most of the problem came from the fake progesterone.

Boy, when that news came out, women were understandably scared—and dropped their HRT. My office was flooded with calls from angry patients who felt duped and afraid, and who were suffering from menopausal symptoms that had returned with a vengeance.

Now we are in a situation in which we know hormones can help some things, including the signs of aging, but may also push cancer buttons we'd prefer not be pushed. Many natural health practitioners consider natural and bioidentical hormones to be much safer. It's believed they do not make the same weird metabolites in our bodies that pregnant horse urine estrogen and synthetic progesterone do. More and more peer-reviewed small-scale studies on bioidentical hormone use are coming out, but large-scale studies have not been completed. While I suspect natural hormones are safer, we cannot be sure.

A 2000 study from the Mayo Clinic looked at 176 postmenopausal women and found that when the women took oral micronized progesterone (a natural form of the hormone), they had much less body pain, fewer hot flashes, and less anxiety and depression. This study showed that the natural hormones did a better job than the synthetic progesterone forms used in conventional gynecological practices. Another, 2008 study comparing natural with conventional supplemental hormones found that the estrogen and natural micronized progesterone had fewer cancer-encouraging effects on breast tissue. This was an observational study, which is not as stringent as the double-blind studies we like to see examining the effects of a drug. (As a side note, I prefer multifactorial to single-drug studies. Multifactorial studies look at diet, lifestyle, and proper supplementation, and therefore treat the person holistically. But if you want to see the effect of purely one substance, then the single-drug paradigm is fine.)

If you are suffering from the signs of aging, and have intense menopausal symptoms, follow the recommendations in this book: work on your sleep, balance your diet, exercise, practice relaxation techniques, and do a nice four-week detox, which will help the liver metabolize your hormones properly. In the majority of my patients who follow this plan, I see reduced menopausal symptoms and no use for supplemental hormones.

If this plan doesn't do the trick, then have blood work done to check your thyroid and adrenal function (using an adrenal saliva stress test) and help get these into balance. Often when the stress system (meaning your adrenal glands along with your brain and nervous system) and thyroid are in working order, the hormones can rebalance.

Low Thyroid?

For low thyroid function that is not caused by inflammatory issues such as Hashimoto's disease (an autoimmune thyroid disorder), I often recommend iodine, tyrosine, and seaweed. If there is an autoimmune issue, go gluten-free and take 200 mcg of selenium to help reduce the inflammation that affects the thyroid. Also, ask yourself if you are holding yourself back from speaking up. According to Dr. Carolyn Myss, Louise Hay, and the ancient systems of body chakras (energy centers), challenges with the throat area and thyroid problems can be a symptom of a woman who does not speak her voice. I have seen this correlation at play many times in my practice.

Adrenal Fatigue?

The adrenal system is responsible for your body's response to stress. The body produces catecholamines (stress hormones), which keep us awake, alert, and responsive. Long-term stress can strain this system and cause it to work suboptimally. This is called adrenal fatigue. The best way to work on it? Get more sleep and lower your stress when you can. Also, I recommend you take a gentle adrenal support supplement, such as my clinic's AdrenAssist, which contains ashwagandha, cordyceps, pantothenic acid (vitamin B_5), and bovine (cow-derived) adrenal gland.

If adrenal and thyroid function are in a better place and you are still not feeling your hormonal best, consider starting natural supplements for estrogen and progesterone *support* (not replacement).

My favorites include chaste berry (also known as vitex) and flax meal. I also use soy foods and a soy isoflavone supplement (50 mg to 150 mg a day), especially if estrogen levels are very low. Isoflavones are phytoestrogens that act by balancing estrogens in the body: When estrogen is low, these gently support estrogen activity. If estrogen is too high, isoflavones will gently lower estrogen activity. Since most premeno-pausal symptoms are due to fluctuating estrogen, us-ing isoflavones can really help. Maca is an herb shown to help with low libido as well.

My Favorite Perimenopausal Supports

If you are having menopausal symptoms—hot flashes, mood changes, and general discomfort—try:

- exercise: will help balance hormones;
- meditation: shown to lower hot flashes by almost half;
- vitamin E (mixed tocopherols): shown to help hot flashes and other symptoms; and
- acupuncture and Chinese herbs: can be miraculous in cases that do not otherwise respond.

How Much Soy Isoflavones in Soy Foods?

Soy food	Isoflavones (mg)	Amount
Cooked soybeans	150	½ cup
Textured soy protein granules	62	¼ cup
Roasted soy nuts	60	¼ cup
Tofu	35	½ cup
Tempeh	35	½ cup
Soy beverage powder	25–75 (varies by manufacturer)	1–2 scoops
Regular soy milk	30	1 cup
Low-fat soy milk	20	1 cup
Roasted soy butter	17	2 tablespoons

If All Else Fails: Natural Hormone Replacement

If the recommendations I've just given are not relieving your symptoms, or the symptoms are unbearable, it may be time to consider natural hormone replacement.

Best to Test

Before starting, test your hormone levels. The best time to test blood estrogen levels is on the third day of menstrual flow. The best day to measure blood progesterone is day twenty-one of a cycle. While it is inconvenient to have your blood taken on two separate days, doing it this way will give you the best indication of your hormone levels. While he or she is testing your blood, have your doctor look at pregnenolone, testosterone, and dehydroepiandrosterone (DHEAs) levels, too. If you are in menopause or not having a regular period thanks to birth control or other factors, don't worry about what day you have your blood drawn.

I also look at urine and saliva hormone tests. No one test is 100 percent accurate, so the best thing is to try all these and then work with a knowledgeable naturopathic doc or other holistic practitioner who can advise you on how to match compounded natural hormones to your particular symptoms, test results, and needs.

Natural hormones are prescribed in oral pill or liquid form, and as creams, suppositories, and subdermal pellets. Typically, these can include estrogen, progesterone, testosterone, and DHEA. If pregnenolone is low, try a replacement first—it is sold over the counter in vitamin shops—to see if it helps relieve symptoms. Pregnenolone is the master molecule from which the other hormones are made. Before starting any hormonal supplement, however, consult a knowledgeable doctor. While these hormones are natural, they need to be used as a last step, once other methods have been tried. And they should be used cautiously, and at the lowest dosage possible.

Chapter 7

SUMMARY AND GLOW CHECKLIST

A goal without a plan is just a wish.

———

—ANTOINE DE SAINT-EXUPÉRY, POET, WRITER,
AND VISIONARY AVIATOR

*W*hew! That was a tour d'health indeed.

Congratulations on making a commitment to your glow. All my patients receive a recommendation plan at the end of every visit. So, here is a template for yours: a quick-reference guide to all the things we've talked about. I want to be sure your plan is clear and in place. Please review the following items, and fill in the spaces with the recommendations you will be using for your own glowing health goals. Take what you have learned from the chapters, especially the parts that resonate with you the most, and note them here, to create your individualized plan.

You may not need to fill this out entirely, and you may not need every step or recommendation. For example, perhaps you don't take supplements at bedtime. Also, you may change the plan over time, as some concerns improve and other challenges become more apparent. That is the way it often works, so be flexible and continue moving forward.

1 ✐ *Beauty Sleep*

Sleep rituals: _____

_____

Bedtime: _____

_____

Supplements for bed:_____

_____

2 ✐ *Beauty Feast*

Water intake:_____

_____

Foods to add:_____

_____

Foods to remove: _____

_____

Mediterranean diet recipes to try: _____

_____

_____

3 ✿ *Move in Your Glow Zone*

Days scheduled and type of exercise: _____

_____

_____

_____

_____

4 ✿ *Inner Peace*

Work on self-esteem: _____

_____

Finding bliss: _____

_____

Helping others: _____

_____

Meditation schedule: _____

_____

Time in nature: _____

_____

Acupuncture: _____

_____

Massage: _____

5 ✍ Spring Cleaning

Plan your four-week week detox: _____

_____

_____

_____

_____

6 ✍ Glowing Remedies

Multiple vitamin: _____

_____

Fish oil: _____

_____

Probiotic:_____

_____

Pycnogenol: _____

_____

Additional remedies based on my needs: _____

_____

_____

_____

Well, there it is. You should be extremely proud of yourself—you have moved through a good deal of information. Have fun being your healthiest and most beautiful, glowing you! Remember, if you need a pep talk, just reread this book.

RESOURCES

Recommended Supplements

....

Ensuring you're taking quality supplements is very important, for government regulation is unfortunately not very good at this time. The supplements mentioned here are those used in our clinic and in the clinics of physicians who search for the highest-quality supplements available. They are all free of allergens and are rigorously tested for contaminants, toxins, and chemicals.

Source I and II Nutrients

A blend of the highest-quality multiple vitamins and minerals, Source I does not contain iron (better for men and postmenopausal women), whereas Source II nutrients contain iron (better for menstruating women).

Ultimate Omega Fish Oil and Cod-Liver Oil

This is an excellent molecularly distilled essential fatty acid.

Restoraflora

This *Lactobacillus* and *Bifidus* combination is used to support optimal digestive health and a balanced microbiome.

AdrenAssist

This Chinese medicine–inspired formulation supports optimal adrenal function.

Melatonin Cadence

This special time-release formula of melatonin helps naturally support best sleep.

Tryptophan Calmplete

Take this tryptophan formulation with B vitamin cofactors for optimal sleep and calming.

Source Cleanse

Our clinic's detox formula, it contains plenty of protein (rice and pea based) along with a quality multiple vitamin, as well as liver and digestion supportive nutrients.

Source Greens

This is the formula I recommend for a greens source. It has chlorella, green tea, astragalus, and a mix of powdered greens, probiotics, and much more, to help aid in detoxification.

Where to Find These

The website **www.3UNeed.com** supplies the same high-quality physician-grade basic multiple vitamin, fish oil, and probiotics that I use in my clinic and take myself. These are all natural and contain no gluten, allergens, cow's milk components, or artificial colors or flavorings. They are also extensively tested during manufacture, from raw material to end product. They are free of contaminants, pesticides, molds, and heavy metals. For full disclosure, please note that this is my website. Of course there are other quality vitamins you can buy. If you prefer not to purchase them here, talk to your naturopathic doctor or other expert to choose the highest-quality supplementation you can find.

Other supplements mentioned in this book can also be found at the Natural Health Store at **www.Inner SourceHealth.com**.

Other Websites I Visit

BeauTeaBar (www.beauteabar.com). My go-to place to buy clean skin-care products and organic makeup.

Environmental Working Group (www.ewg.org). An excellent unbiased resource regarding toxin research and guides to purchasing clean, nontoxic products.

Worlds Healthiest Foods (www.whfoods.com). A noncommercial repository of top-quality research on the nutritional value of foods.

Books I Love

....

Clean, Green, and Lean: Get Rid of the Toxins That Make You Fat (Wiley). Written by my environmental medicine teacher, Dr. Walter Crinnion, one of the world's top experts on toxins and disease.

Eat Right for Your Blood Type: The Individualized Diet Solution (Penguin). This landmark book describes how to use blood type to address your health. Written by Dr. Peter D'Adamo, one of the smartest physicians on the planet.

The Encyclopedia of Natural Medicine (Prima Publishing). A reference that should be on everyone's shelf. Written by Dr. Michael Murray and Dr. Joseph Pizzorno, this is the go-to naturopathic guide for virtually every condition.

Put Anxiety Behind You: The Complete Drug-Free Program (Red Wheel/Conari Press). My husband, Peter, wrote this book. It has helped scores of people conquer their anxiety.

How Come They're Happy and I'm Not? The Complete Natural Program for Healing Depression for Good, Peter's other book, tackles the issue of depression. Find both books on Amazon or visit www.drpeterbongiorno.com.

Books with Positive Messages

Creative Visualization, by Shakti Gawain.

The Power of Now, by Eckhart Tolle.

A Return to Love, by Marianne Williamson.

Sacred Contracts, by Caroline Myss.

When Things Fall Apart, by Pema Chödrön.

Where to Find Natural Medicine Practitioners

American Association of Naturopathic Physicians (www.naturopathic.org). This website lists only accredited naturopathic physicians well trained in proper naturopathic medical schools. Also, consider supporting the licensing of naturopathic doctors in the state of New York by visiting the website of the New York Association of Naturopathic Physicians at www .NYANP.org.

Surviving Mold (www.survivingmold.com). This website is based on the work of Dr. Ritchie

Shoemaker, who pioneered the protocol to help diagnose mold sensitivity and treat it properly.

National Certification Commission for Acupuncturists (www.nccaom.org).

The American Massage Therapy Association (www. amtamassage.org).

For Other Products

....

Multipure (www.multipure.com) for high-quality water filters.

IQAir (www.iqair.com) for high-quality air filters.

CONTACT INFORMATION FOR
DR. PINA LOGIUDICE

Practices at Inner Source Health, with offices in
New York (Long Island and New York City)

Personal website: www.DrPinaND.com

Clinic website: www.InnerSourceHealth.com

Twitter: @drpinaND

E-mail: info@innersourcehealth.com

Phone: (631) 421-1848

ACKNOWLEDGMENTS

First, I would like to acknowledge and thank God for my life. I have been so blessed, and I'm in ever-loving gratitude.

I would also like to acknowledge my parents, Sebastiano and Carmela LoGiudice, for giving me my foundation and support. There aren't enough words to express my gratitude and love. To my family, the Cioffis, LoGiudices, and Bongiornos, thank you for being who you are in my life.

To Katharine Sands, my agent at Sarah Jane Freymann Literary Agency, and Jeanette Shaw, my editor at Tarcher Perigee, thank you for believing in this project; and thanks to Toni Robino for being a compass in guiding me through.

To Dr. Peter Bongiorno, my amazing husband. This book would not have been possible without you. Your guidance is steady, your compassion is sincere, and your love profound. Thank you for all that you are. I love you with all that I am.

For Sophia, for the wisest, sweetest soul I know. Thank you for bringing your light to this world.

REFERENCES

Introduction

Bishop, K. S., and L. R. Ferguson. "The Interaction Between Epigenetics, Nutrition and the Development of Cancer." *Nutrients* 7, no. 2 (2015): 922–47.

Ho, S. M. et al. "Environmental Epigenetics and Its Implication on Disease Risk and Health Outcomes." *ILAR Journal* 53, no. 3–4 (2012): 289–305.

Olshansky, S. J. et al. "A Potential Decline in Life Expectancy in the United States in the Twenty-First Century." *New England Journal of Medicine* 352, no. 11 (2005): 1138–45.

Chapter 1: *Your Beauty Sleep*

Abdou, A. M. et al. "Relaxation and Immunity Enhancement Effects of Gamma-Aminobutyric Acid

(GABA) Administration in Humans." *Biofactors* 26, no. 3 (2006): 201–8.

Demisch, K. et al. "Treatment of Severe Chronic Insomnia with L-tryptophan: Results of a Double-Blind Cross-Over Study." *Pharmacopsychiatry* 20, no. 6 (1987): 242–44.

Kaviani, N. et al. The Efficacy of *Passiflora incarnata linnaeus* in Reducing Dental Anxiety in Patients Undergoing Periodontal Treatment." *Journal of Dentistry* 14, no. 2 (2013): 68–72.

Kripke, D. F. et al. "Hypnotics' Association with Mortality or Cancer: A Matched Cohort Study." *British Medical Journal* 2, no. 1 (2012): e000850. doi: 10.1136/bmjopen-2012-000850.

Chapter 2: Food and Digestion

Akesson, A. et al. "Low-Risk Diet and Lifestyle Habits in the Primary Prevention of Myocardial Infarction in Men: A Population-Based Prospective Cohort Study." *Journal of the American College of Cardiology* 64, no. 13 (2014): 1299–306.

Bland, J. *The Disease Delusion*. New York: Harper Collins, 2014, p. 242.

REFERENCES

Bonaccio, M. et al. "Mediterranean Diet and Low-Grade Subclinical Inflammation: The Moli-Sani Study." *Endocrine, Metabolic, and Immune Disorders—Drug Targets* 15, no. 1 (2015): 18–24.

Buettner, D. *The Blue Zones: 9 Lessons for Living Longer.* Washington, DC: National Geographic Society, 2008.

Bunch, T. J. et al. "Association of Body Weight with Total Mortality and with ICD Shocks Among Survivors of Ventricular Fibrillation in Out-of-Hospital Cardiac Arrest." *Resuscitation* 77, no. 3 (2008): 351–55.

Cooper, C. et al. "Modifiable Predictors of Dementia in Mild Cognitive Impairment: A Systematic Review and Meta-analysis." *American Journal of Psychiatry* 173, no. 4 (2015): 323–34.

Gaby, A. R. *Nutritional Medicine.* Concord, NH: Fritz Perlberg Publishing, 2010, pp. 1323–26.

Iwasaki, M. et al. "Plasma Isoflavone Level and Subsequent Risk of Breast Cancer Among Japanese Women: A Nested Case-Control Study from the Japan Public Health Center-Based Prospective Study Group." *Journal of Clinical Oncology* 26, no. 10 (2008): 1677–83.

Rondanelli, M. et al. "Satiety and Amino Acid Profile in Overweight Women After a New Treatment Using a Natural Plant Extract Sublingual Spray Formulation." *International Journal of Obesity* 33, no. 10 (2009): 1174–82.

Toledo, E. et al. "Mediterranean Diet and Invasive Breast Cancer Risk Among Women at High Cardiovascular Risk in the PREDIMED Trial: A Randomized Clinical Trial." *JAMA Internal Medicine* 175, no. 11 (2015): 1752–60.

Uribarri, J. et al. "Diet-Derived Advanced Glycation End Products Are Major Contributors to the Body's AGE Pool and Induce Inflammation in Healthy Subjects." *Annals of the New York Academy of Sciences* 1043 (2005): 461–66.

Wu, Y. C. et al. "Meta-analysis of Studies on Breast Cancer Risk and Diet in Chinese Women." *International Journal of Clinical and Experimental Medicine* 8, no. 1 (2015): 73–85.

Chapter 3: Move in Your Glow Zone

Kim, J. et al. "The Effects of Physical Activity on Breast Cancer Survivors After Diagnosis." *Journal of Cancer Prevention* 18, no. 3 (2013): 193–200.

REFERENCES

Reynolds, G. "Younger Skin Through Exercise." *New York Times*, April 16, 2014.

Schnohr, P. et al. "Dose of Jogging and Long-Term Mortality: The Copenhagen City Heart Study." *Journal of American College of Cardiology* 65, no. 5 (2015): 411–19.

Winters-Stone, K. M. et al. "Strength Training Stops Bone Loss and Builds Muscle in Postmenopausal Breast Cancer Survivors: A Randomized, Controlled Trial." *Breast Cancer Research and Treatment* 127, no. 2 (2011): 447–56.

Zhou, J. et al. "A Meta-Analysis on the Efficacy of Tai Chi in Patients with Parkinson's Disease Between 2008 and 2014." *Evidence-Based Complementary and Alternative Medicine* 593 (2015): 263.

Chapter 4: Relaxation and Inner Peace

Epel, E. et al. "Can Meditation Slow Rate of Cellular Aging? Cognitive Stress, Mindfulness, and Telomeres." *Annals of New York Academy of Sciences* 1172 (August 2009): 34–53.

Moyer, Christopher A. et al. "A Meta-Analysis of Massage Therapy Research." *Psychological Bulletin* 130, no. 1 (2004): 3–18.

Chapter 5: Detoxification

Andrade, J. P., and M. Assunção. "Protective Effects of Chronic Green Tea Consumption on Age-Related Neurodegeneration." *Current Pharmaceutical Design* 18, no. 1 (2012): 4–14.

Arslan, G. G., and I. Eşer. "An Examination of the Effect of Castor Oil Packs on Constipation in the Elderly." *Complementary Therapeutic Clinical Practice* 17, no. 1 (2011): 58–62.

Emmanuel, A. V. et al. "Relationship Between Psychological State and Level of Activity of Extrinsic Gut Innervation in Patients with a Functional Gut Disorder." *Gut* 49, no. 2 (2001): 209–13.

Environmental Protection Agency. Chloroform Hazard Summary. http://www.epa.gov/ttnatw01/hlthef/chlorofo.html.

Flora, S. J. et al. "Prevention of Arsenic Induced Hepatic Apoptosis by Concomitant Administration of Garlic Extracts in Mice." *Chemico-Biological Interactions* 177, no. 3 (2008): 227–33.

Houston, M. C. "Role of Mercury Toxicity in Hypertension, Cardiovascular Disease, and Stroke."

REFERENCES

Journal of Clinical Hypertension 13, no. 8 (2011): 621–27.

Jedrychowski, W., and U. Maugeri. "An Apple a Day May Hold Colorectal Cancer at Bay: Recent Evidence from a Case-Control Study." *Reviews on Environmental Health* 24, no. 1 (2009): 59–74.

Kharb S. et al. "Fluoride Levels and Osteosarcoma." *South Asian Journal of Cancer* 1, no. 2 (2012): 76–77.

Ko, R. J. et al. "Adulterants in Asian Patent Medicines." *New England Journal of Medicine* 339, no. 12 (1998): 847.

Kumar, J. V. "The Association Between Enamel Fluorosis and Dental Caries in U.S. Schoolchildren." *Journal of the American Dental Association* 14D, no. 7 (2009).

Lee, D. H. et al. "A Strong Dose-Response Relation Between Serum Concentrations of Persistent Organic Pollutants and Diabetes: Results from the National Health and Examination Survey, 1999–2002." *Diabetes Care* 29, no. 7 (2006): 1638–44.

Navarrete-Solís, J. et al. "A Double-Blind, Randomized Clinical Trial of Niacinamide 4% versus

REFERENCES

Hydroquinone 4% in the Treatment of Melasma."
Dermatology Research and Practice 379 (2011): 173. doi:
10.1155/2011/379173.

Panossian, A. "Effects of Adaptogens on the Central
Nervous System and the Molecular Mechanisms
Associated with Their Stress—Protective Activity."
Pharmaceuticals 3, no. 1 (2010): 188–224.

Saper, R. B. et al. "Heavy Metal Content of Ayurvedic
Herbal Medicine Products." *JAMA* 292, no. 23 (2004):
2868–73.

Sorrentino, J. A. et al. "Defining the Toxicology of
Aging." *Trends in Molecular Medicine* 20, no. 7 (2014):
375–84.

Starfield, B. "Is US Health Really the Best in the
World?" *JAMA* 284, no. 4 (2000): 483–85.

Vieira Senger, A. E. et al. "Effect of Green Tea
(*Camellia sinensis*) Consumption on the Components of
Metabolic Syndrome in Elderly." *Journal of Nutrition
Health and Aging* 16, no. 9 (2012): 738–42.

Water Authority of Great Neck North. "Fluoridation
Not Necessary," 2007. http://www.waterauthorityof
greatnecknorth.com/fluoridation_not_necessary.html.

REFERENCES

Zhang, J., R. Stewart, M. Phillips, Q. Shi, and M. Prince. "Pesticide Exposure and Suicidal Ideation in Rural Communities in Zhejiang Province, China." *Bulletin of the World Health Organization* 87, no. 10 (2009): 745–53.

Chapter 6: Glowing Supplements and Hormonal Harmony

Bailey, R. L. et al. "Multivitamin-Mineral Use Is Associated with Reduced Risk of Cardiovascular Disease Mortality Among Women in the United States." *Journal of Nutrition* 145, no. 3 (2015): 572–78.

Buckshee, K., D. Takkar, and N. Aggarwal. "Micronized Flavonoid Therapy in Internal Hemorrhoids of Pregnancy." *International Journal of Gynecology and Obstetrics* 57, no. 2 (1997): 145–51.

Chiu, A. E. et al. "Double-Blinded, Placebo-Controlled Trial of Green Tea Extracts in the Clinical and Histologic Appearance of Photoaging Skin." *Dermatologic Surgery* 31, no. 7, Part 2 (2005): 855–60.

Cho, S. et al. "Dietary Aloe Vera Supplementation Improves Facial Wrinkles and Elasticity and It Increases the Type I Procollagen Gene Expression in

Human Skin in Vivo." *Annals of Dermatology* 21, no. 1 (2009): 6–11.

ConsumerLab. "Probiotics Review: Probiotics (for Adults, Children and Pets) and Kefirs." https://www.consumerlab.com/reviews/Probiotic_Supplements_Lactobacillus_acidophilus_Bifidobacterium/probiotics/#results.

Davis, D. R. et al. "Changes in USDA Food Composition Data for 43 Garden Crops, 1950 to 1999." *Journal of the American College of Nutrition* 23, no. 6 (2004): 669–82.

DermNet NZ. "Polypodium leucotomos." http://www.dermnetnz.org/treatments/polypodium.html.

Fitzpatrick, L. A. et al. "Comparison of Regimens Containing Oral Micronized Progesterone or Medroxyprogesterone Acetate on Quality of Life in Postmenopausal Women: A Cross-Sectional Survey." *Journal of Women's Health and Gender-Based Medicine* 9, no. 4 (2000): 381–87.

Fournier, A. et al. "Use of Different Postmenopausal Hormone Therapies and Risk of Histology- and Hormone Receptor–Defined Invasive Breast Cancer." *Journal of Clinical Oncology* 26, no. 8 (2008): 1260–68.

REFERENCES

Frank, E. et al. "Use of Vitamin-Mineral Supplements by Female Physicians in the United States." *American Journal of Clinical Nutrition* 72, no. 4 (2000): 969–75.

Gärtner, R. "Selenium Supplementation in Patients with Autoimmune Thyroiditis Decreases Thyroid Peroxidase Antibodies Concentrations." *Journal of Clinical Endocrinology and Metabolism* 87, no. 4 (2002): 1687–91.

Glossmann, H. "Vitamin D, UV, and Skin Cancer in the Elderly: To Expose or Not to Expose?" *Gerontology* 57, no. 4 (2011): 350–53.

Hardell, L., and M. Carlberg. "Mobile Phone and Cordless Phone Use and the Risk for Glioma—Analysis of Pooled Case-Control Studies in Sweden, 1997–2003 and 2007–2009." *Pathophysiology* 22, no. 1 (2015): 1–13.

Harris, E. et al. "The Effect of Multivitamin Supplementation on Mood and Stress in Healthy Older Men." *Human Psychopharmacology* 26, no. 8 (2011): 560–67.

McCormack, D. and D. McFadden. "A Review of Pterostilbene Antioxidant Activity and Disease Modification." *Oxidative Medicine and Cellular Longevity* 575 (2013): 482.

REFERENCES

McDaniel, J. C. et al. "Fish Oil Supplementation Alters Levels of Lipid Mediators of Inflammation in Microenvironment of Acute Human Wounds." *Wound Repair and Regeneration* 19, no. 2 (2011): 189–200.

Metchnikoff, E. *The Prolongation of Life: Optimistic Studies.* New York: G. P. Putnam's Sons, 1910), p. 96.

Misner, B. "Food Alone May Not Provide Sufficient Micronutrients for Preventing Deficiency." *Journal of the International Society of Sports Nutrition* 3, no. 1 (2006): 51–55.

Pandiri, A. R. et al. "Aloe Vera Non-Decolorized Whole Leaf Extract–Induced Large Intestinal Tumors in F344 Rats Share Similar Molecular Pathways with Human Sporadic Colorectal Tumors." *Toxicologic Pathology* 39, no. 7 (2011): 1065–74.

Pizzorno, J. "Naturopathic Principles." Keynote speech at the 2010 AANP Convention. Portland, OR, August 2010.

Rossouw, J. E. et al. "Risks and Benefits of Estrogen Plus Progestin in Healthy Postmenopausal Women: Principal Results from the Women's Health Initiative Randomized Controlled Trial." *JAMA* 288, no. 3 (2002): 321–33.

REFERENCES

Tominaga, K. et al. "Cosmetic Benefits of Astaxanthin on Humans Subjects." *Acta Biochimica Polonica* 59, no. 1 (2012): 43–47.

Verdier-Sévrain, S. "Effect of Estrogens on Skin Aging and the Potential Role of Selective Estrogen Receptor Modulators." *Climacteric* 10, no. 4 (2007): 289–97.

Xu, Q. et al. "Multivitamin Use and Telomere Length in Women." *American Journal of Clinical Nutrition* 89, no. 6 (2009): 1857–63.